Clinical Documentation for Mental Health Clinicians

INTRODUCTION OF SERVICE TO DISCHARGE AND EVERYTHING IN BETWEEN

Mona Gallo, Editor

Lindsey Wilson College

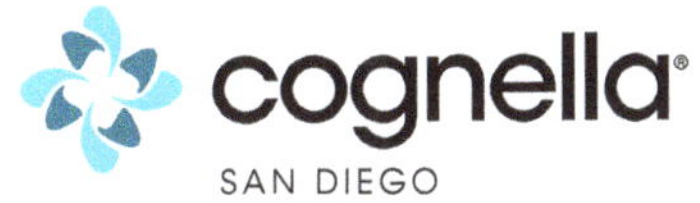

Bassim Hamadeh, CEO and Publisher
Amy Smith, Associate Editorial Manager
Abbey Hastings, Senior Production Editor
Emely Villavicencio, Senior Graphic Designer
Kylie Bartolome, Licensing Specialist
Natalie Piccotti, Director of Marketing
Kassie Graves, Senior Vice President, Editorial
Alia Bales, Director, Project Editorial and Production

Printed in the United States of America.

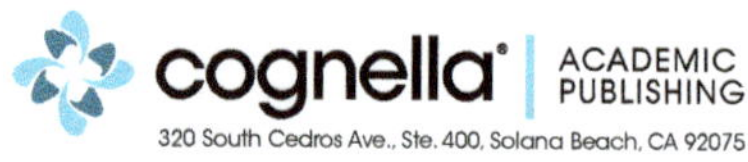

BRIEF CONTENTS

DETAILED CONTENTS

Acknowledgments

As the primary author, I wanted to express my deepest gratitude to the talented group of authors who joined me to write this compilation of research and experience. In some instances, preexisting literature has very little to nothing to say regarding specific portions of a client file. While there may be some vacancies, these authors have helped to fill in some of the gaps in the literature by sharing their professional experiences in multiple additions and examples provided in this book.

Primary author:

Mona Gallo, EdD, LPCC-S
Associate Professor of Counseling
Lindsey Wilson College

Contributing authors:

Gregory L. Bohner PhD, LPC-MHSP, CCMHC
Assistant Professor
Lindsey Wilson College

Keeley Stewart, PhD
Assistant Professor
Lindsey Wilson College

Darlene Vaughn, PhD., CSAC, NCC, LPCC
Assistant Professor
Lindsey Wilson College

Marisa L. White, PhD, LPC
Associate Professor
Lindsey Wilson College

Holly J. Mattingly, PhD
Assistant Professor
Lindsey Wilson College

Melinda Mays, EdD, LPCC-S, NCC
Associate Professor
Lindsey Wilson College

Daniel R. Romero, PhD, LPCC-S, NCC
Associate Professor
Lindsey Wilson College

CHAPTER 1

The Purpose of Clinical Documentation

Mona Gallo, EdD, Holly J. Mattingly, PhD, Daniel R. Romero, PhD, Darlene Vaughn, PhD, and Gregory L. Bohner, PhD

This book has been generated because of the professional expectation for clinicians to be competent in the area of documentation, as well as the reported general lack of literature guiding clinicians through the clinical documentation process (Kodweis et al., 2021; Prieto & Scheel, 2002). Instructors are offered guidance in the presentation of the material to students, and students gain an initial understanding of concepts and will master them as they connect them to the content of this and the remaining chapters.

This chapter will examine the need for clinical documentation in counseling, including the history of documentation, ethical and legal reasons for documentation, documentation for insurance purposes, industry expectations, and how to be clear and concise in clinical reporting. Clinical documentation occurs throughout the entirety of a client's counseling involvement and is used to record the entirety of client contact. This process begins with the initial contact of the client, carries on throughout treatment, and includes any provisions through discharge from treatment. Sometimes, contact may continue even after the client's discharge. There are many categories of clinical documentation, such as identifying or intake information. There is also a case conceptualization that includes a great deal of data such as vocational/educational, spiritual, drug, alcohol, and medical assessments. Clinical documentation also includes individualized treatment plans, case notes, and other documentation such as releases of information, communications from stakeholders, results of tests/assessments, and discharge or termination documentation (Piazza & Baruth, 1990). Each chapter of this textbook distinctly addresses the main pieces of documentation a clinician may utilize during their training and career. This textbook leads the reader through the informed consent process, release of information, an intake/assessment, the case conceptualization, case notes, and the discharge/termination summary, as well as crisis documentation.

INTRODUCTION

Clinical documentation has long been a part of any kind of medical treatment, including the treatment of mental and emotional disorders. Too often, mental health practitioners have learned how to document their interactions with clients while "on the job," through a practicum/internship training and in postgraduate field experience. Plenty of clinicians have felt sorely underprepared about producing ethically and legally sound clinical documentation that would also meet the demands of insurance providers and withstand legal review.

Over time, clinicians have encountered an increasing demand for required clinical documentation, as well as the need to meet the expectations for their effectiveness in identifying and resolving the client's presenting concerns. Many of these expectations are part of agency policies, budget, and managed care. Managed care companies, and consumers alike, expect to be informed of the anticipated number of sessions that would be necessary to resolve the client's presenting concerns, as well as interventions that could be incorporated into treatment.

Clinicians are expected to provide the consumer and the managed care company with a variety of services. These service expectations frequently include providing stakeholders with an accurate diagnosis, a thorough treatment plan that proposes clearly defined goals, objectives, and specific interventions, reports of any crisis intervention, case management support, and thorough discharge planning. The expectation is that services will be researched, aligned with a theory, and concisely and thoroughly documented.

While the clinician is being trained, they need to develop a knowledge base related to interpreting client cases and producing clinical documentation for said cases. Development of this knowledge base helps to guide the learner through the problem-solving process in the identification and understanding of clients' case documentation and hone their ability to transfer this practice knowledge to new client case situations. Kodweis et al. (2021) noted that the best outcome for a clinician in training is found in both providing the clinician in training with completed case documentation examples and then the opportunity to have them practice their acquired knowledge in completing client case documentation on their own. To support both learning opportunities, each chapter of this textbook provides a thorough example of documentation on two different client cases from two different theoretical approaches.

THE NEED FOR CLINICAL DOCUMENTATION

Prior to the 20th century, cases were only documented for teaching purposes (Decker et al., 2023). It was not until the 1930s that clinicians began documenting practices for client care (Bertolote, 2008). At this time the United States National Committee for Mental Hygiene aimed to fulfill its mission by working jointly with governmental and private institutions that impact the field of mental health. Their mission included supporting early diagnosis and treatment, developing appropriate inpatient support, and providing education to individuals and groups in the personal application of mental health essentials (Bertolote, 2008). As the movement toward improving psychiatric care evolved, so did the need for clear, adequate, and accurate clinical documentation.

Outside of legal, ethical, and insurance purposes, there are many reasons clinicians use clinical documentation. Documentation can assist clinicians in thoughtfully recording observations, patterns, and clients' and other stakeholders' reported data. Providing an intake interview or collecting data from intake documentation along with any assessments can provide a clinician with a starting point in understanding a client's presenting problems and maladaptive patterns (Sperry, 2022). Accurate clinical documentation can assist a clinician in providing a continuity of care to the client, as well as serve as a means of communication to other professionals in the field (Gutheil & Hilliard, 2001). Accurate clinical documentation may also be the only evidence to defend a clinician in an ethical or legal investigation (Health Providers Service Organization [HPSO], 2019).

HISTORY OF CLINICAL DOCUMENTATION

Literature on the history of clinical documentation in counseling is scant. Mental health clinical documentation evolved from the history of medical records (Prieto & Scheel, 2002). In their book on the history of medical records, Lorkowski and Pokorski (2022) define *medical records* as documents that indicate an identified person being treated and include the person's health history, clinical symptoms, diagnostic and treatment process, including medications used and the reason for their use, and a follow-up with the identified patient. These authors note that the earliest medical records found appear in pictorials. In the United States, medical records were first recorded in the Book of Admissions and the Book of Discharges in the New York Hospital in 1793 (Lorkowski & Polorski, 2022, p. 5). This was the birth of the modern record-keeping system, and records were neither organized nor correlated to specific individuals. Early in the 20th century, the mental health field was emerging (Bertolote, 2008), and at the same time, individual records began to evolve with practitioners recording patient data in a single record that was coordinated by the individual's specific identifying information. This construct of a record-keeping system continued to evolve into what we are more accustomed to today (Lorkowski & Polorski, 2022).

In the 1960s, digital health records were introduced, but data entry consisted of transferring information from paper documents to digital records. This system was chaotic, time-consuming, and tedious. As of 2022, about 80% of medical care systems use digital record-keeping platforms to document treatment, procedures, investigation, and analysis (Lorkowski & Pokorski, 2022). Most recently, artificial intelligence has been aiding practitioners in cultivating "the practice of evidence-based medicine, assisting with diagnosis and treatment, helping predict pandemic outbreaks, and reducing medical errors" (Lorkowski & Pokorski, 2022, p. 8).

The continued evolution from paper-based records to digital records has assisted in clinical services being more manageable, more directed toward prevention, and increasingly cost-effective (Lorkowski & Pokorski, 2022). Not only does the practitioner benefit from streamlined records but the patient also has a better opportunity to receive more targeted and effective care.

ETHICAL REASONS FOR CLINICAL DOCUMENTATION

All the predominant mental health professions have a code of ethics to guide clinicians in their professional behavior. Each mental health profession also provides guiding principles that oversee the purpose, use of, and recommendations for record keeping. Overall, the guiding principles are similar to one another, no matter the organizational division of mental health practice: Veracity in clinical documentation is imperative as a means of demonstrating fair and just choices and behaviors in client treatment options, professional choices, and when working in conjunction with other professionals. Thorough and accurate clinical documentation assists in demonstrating that a clinician is practicing with nonmaleficence and beneficence while treating clients. Concise clinical documentation exhibits the clinician's fidelity to the clients who receive services and to the other professionals involved in treatment. Lastly, thorough clinical documentation can demonstrate a client's autonomy in treatment and the decisions to control the direction of their own life choices. The depth and breadth of ethical guidance, however, varies depending on the professional organization.

The American Counseling Association's ([ACA], 2014) *2014 ACA Code of Ethics* denotes a clinician who is practicing as a counselor works in conjunction with the client to develop, maintain, review, and revise a plan that assists the client in reaching reasonable goals, all while honoring the client's freedom of choice. The clinician is guided to create appropriate treatment documents that depict the need for the service. Clinicians are directed to accurately document the client's progress and the services provided. These plans are to match the client's developmental level while considering the client's proficiency and circumstances (ACA, 2014).

In contemporary counseling settings, any referral and screening documentation initiates the development of the client record, including demographic information (Whiston, 2017). Demographics usually include the client's name, contact information, marital status, date of birth, and guardian information and may also include insurer, referral source, and supportive collateral sources (Ivey et al., 2018; Sheparis et al., 2017). Many additional pieces of information are collected during the intake process: phone number(s), including indication of whether a message can be left and on which voicemail, physical street address, sex, next of kin, emergency contact person, current people the client is residing with, employment status, date and reason for organizational engagement, and current and previous mental and physical health providers (Baird, 2005). In addition, many organizations require potential clients to provide copies of identification materials and insurance, financial, or court documents.

The *2014 ACA Code of Ethics* (ACA, 2014) also guides clinicians to disclose to clients when they are working as part of an interdisciplinary treatment team. These treatment teams may include supervised trainees along with other professionals. The client's documentation would include references to the treatment team, what information may be shared between which treatment team members, and the rationale for sharing the information. Clinicians are required to protect client documentation. Safeguarding client documentation includes limiting access to clinical documents by authorized providers who are part of the client's treatment team. In some circumstances, these authorized providers may only have access to portions of the case file documents that are relevant to the services they are providing for the client. Whether the clinician is working alone or as part of a treatment team, clinicians are required to safeguard the client's clinical documents in any medium (ACA, 2014).

The National Association of Social Workers' ([NASW], 2021) *Code of Ethics of the National Association of Social Workers* indicates a clinician practicing as a social worker should take appropriate precautions to document client services accurately, limiting information that is documented to relevant services that are provided. Supporting the concept of consistency in care, clinicians are to adhere to documenting client care in a sufficient and timely manner, whether services are continuing with the current clinician or a future service provider (NASW, 2021).

The American Psychological Association's ([APA], 2017) *Ethical Principles of Psychologists and Code of Conduct* denotes a clinician practicing as a psychologist has a primary responsibility to implement safeguards to protect confidential client information, no matter the medium used. These clinicians are expected to create, maintain, store, share, and dispose of clinical documentation within their control while adhering to any institutional or legal requirements. They are required to document the client's agreement or lack thereof in services. Supporting the concept of consistency in care, clinicians who are psychologists are directed to document thoroughly to provide current or future client care whether by themselves or a different provider. When client documentation is in a shared system, clinicians must avoid documenting personal information that may clearly identify the client and use coding information as needed (APA, 2017).

LEGAL REASONS FOR CLINICAL DOCUMENTATION

According to a report by HPSO (2019), clinicians need to know and adhere to requirements set forth by their specific state practice laws and regulations, the industry standards of care, policies of the licensing board, as well as the policies of their agency. When there are multiple requirements that are set forth by any of the aforementioned information sources, then the clinician should comply with the most "stringent policy" (Barnett et al., 2014; HPSO, 2019, p. 2).

Clinical documentation should be thorough, accurate, objective, and current, demonstrating support to the client's treatment, and satisfy a state's licensing board statutes (HPSO, 2019). So, how thorough is thorough? Clinicians should document

> the clinical decision-making process, as well as the client's diagnosis, service plan, response to treatment, results of diagnostic testing and/or consultation findings, and assessments of the client's risk of being a danger to self or others [in addition to] client education regarding the client's treatment agreement, and education regarding policies and procedures. (HPSO, 2021, p. 4).

Recommendations for thorough clinical documentation must meet many minimal requirements. According to the Health Insurance Portability and Accountability Act (HIPAA) of 1996, health care providers should maintain a "designated record set" that clients have a right to access. A *designated record set* is defined as records concerning individuals' medical and billing information, which are either managed by or on behalf of a health care provider subject to regulations, systems containing enrollment, payment, claims adjudication, and case or medical management records, managed by or for a health plan. Additionally, this includes any records employed, either wholly or partially, by or for the covered entity in the decision-making process concerning individuals. This encompasses records utilized for decision-making about any individuals, irrespective of whether they have been specifically used for the individual seeking access (Modifications to HIPAA Privacy, Security, Enforcement, and Breach Notification Rules, 2013).

It is suggested for the clinician to always include the service date and time in data entry and to gain informed consent from the client before treatment and testing—and to record it. Clinicians are to document any and all discussions with the client that address privacy, confidentiality, and potential exceptions to these protections. They are expected to document any outside session contact (e.g., phone, email, fax, etc.) with the client and/or other stakeholders, including the person spoken to, clinical advice given, and any actions executed. It is further suggested clinicians are responsible to record any resources that may enhance the treatment process that were provided to the client.

Documentation about assessments or evaluations needs to include the date and time of the assessment, results of the evaluation, and the duration that such conclusions are valid. The clinician should record when referrals or consultations were made, including an explanation of additional actions carried out. For clients who are referred for psychotropic treatment, the clinician should also document current prescriptions and who is monitoring the client for medication compliance. Documentation in the client's file may also include any signs that the client is unwilling or unable to adhere to the agreements made in treatment, such as missing appointments, refusals to supply data, or recommendation rejections. The documentation also incorporates efforts made by the clinician to follow up with the client and any attempts to educate the client regarding risks in not cooperating or declining treatment options. Clinical session notes often reflect any review of and changes regarding the client's problems and treatment plan, as well as the client's response to any of the changes. If there is an error in the clinical documentation, the clinician does not alter entries. Instead, the clinician may use an addendum and thoroughly notate that it is an addendum to the clinical document, or the clinician can use a strikethrough on the error on the original document and initial the strikethrough. Either the addendum or strikethrough would be dated, signed, and kept with the unedited initial document to retain that entry and original date (Erford, 2015; HPSO, 2019).

Thorough documentation is an essential ingredient to aid a clinician in avoiding detrimental legal actions and complaints filed with a licensing board. Thorough, accurate, objective, and current clinical documentation can offer the strongest defense against legal or ethical board actions against the clinician. During a legal investigation, the clinical documentation is the documented support and accounts of the clinician and may become the only item of evidence in a defense (Erford, 2015; Gutheil & Hilliard, 2001; HPSO, 2019). It should be noted that psychotherapy notes by the clinician, also referred to as *process notes*, are specifically excluded from the designated record set required by federal law. *Psychotherapy notes* are considered the personal notes made by the clinician analyzing the subject matter of the therapy session and are kept separate from the client's designated record set (U.S. Department of Health and Human Services, 2022).

Professional organizations have directed the creation and maintenance of clinical case records for years, but the enactment of HIPAA created a national framework for security and confidentiality for health care data and information (Zhang & Parsons, 2016). HIPAA stipulates professional behaviors related to documentation, such as the maintenance of written or electronic HIPAA policies and procedures, as well as maintenance of written records related to client service needs as outlined in HIPAA (Zhang & Parsons, 2016). HIPAA has a requirement for periodic review of the documentation and permits document destruction after 6 years from its creation or from the last service date (Zhang & Parsons, 2016). Following both HIPAA mandates and state laws on documentation is a common expectation for all clinical counseling practitioners.

USE OF CLEAR AND CONCISE LANGUAGE IN CLINICAL DOCUMENTATION

In addition to rule and law adherence, it is essential for clinicians to document all professional engagement and any client assessment in an explicit, truthful, and objective manner that is void of jargon, biased language, and irrelevant details (ACA, 2014; NASW, 2021). Clarity in clinical documentation is both a deliberate and a conscious choice. The clinician makes a concerted effort to choose what clinical data will be documented and how they will document it. Clinicians must also reserve enough time to produce timely and accurate clinical documentation (Erford, 2015). It is also best practice for a clinician to choose a professional documentation style that they maintain throughout the client's case file, as well as from case to case.

Clarity of language in clinical documentation can assist the clinician of record and any other professionals who are viewing or referring to a client's documentation. Clinicians must consider the audience who will read the documentation and write to that audience (Baird, 2005). Documenting clearly can support the clinician and other adjunct providers in considering alternate diagnoses, the basis of the client's problems, and plans for treatment (Falvey et al., 2005; Zhang & Parsons, 2016).

Clinicians need to remember that their writing should be crafted to the reader, not the author. In considering the audience, ask yourself, is the reader a third-party payer, a legal professional, a medical professional, another clinician, a treatment team member, or the client themselves? Considering the audience will guide the clinician's style of communication (Baird, 2005). In addition to evaluating the words chosen in recording clinical data, clinicians also choose the amount of words to document clinical data (Baird, 2005). More is not always better. Clear data that summarizes the event in a brief and concise way is better than muddled data that lacks clarity, is indiscernible to the audience, or may imply information that was not intended. Once the entry is documented, the clinician may not be available to explain the data. Clinicians must exercise caution, write with clarity, and use a dictionary when necessary. The use of clear and concise language may reduce potential misunderstandings and misinterpretations of data.

Clarity in clinical documentation allows the clinician to only report relative case details that focus specifically on the client. Clear clinical documentation will delineate between what the client reported and what the clinician observed. Clinicians document any assessments provided, the scores or interpretation of the client's scores, as well as any clinical recommendations and specific referrals (Zhang & Parsons, 2016). It is best practice to document the client's diagnosis(es), differential diagnosis(es), the rationale for the diagnosis(es), use of a provisional diagnosis(es), or lack of a diagnosis. It is also exceptionally important to clearly document the plan for treatment, what the client agreed to or refused to do, as well as how the clinician followed up with the client on any agreed-upon plans or homework. Clinicians should regularly review the client's file to follow up with the client on what has been achieved and what still needs to be addressed. The clinician needs to document the process performed to track any outstanding tasks, recommendations, interventions, and referrals (Zhang & Parsons, 2016).

The specific language used in clinical documentation is important. Clinicians must balance providing necessary information while also protecting the client. This balance is more than just the amount of information shared; it also includes the type of information written and even use of specific terms. This is particularly important with client identifiers. To protect the client, it is essential that clinicians document in a way that is sensitive to the lived experience of the client (Decker et al., 2023). Writing statements made by the client is acceptable and encouraged. Placing a client's statements in quotation marks allows a reader an opportunity in awareness that may not be otherwise apparent. The responsibility for clinicians to protect the client can be complicated; for example, the client may want documentation to identify them with gender-fluid terminology. While this may seem appropriate because doing so could influence rapport and trust with the client, it is important to think about other impacts. For example, using specific identifiers could put the client at risk of discrimination should the documentation be viewed by others, such as collaborative professionals, courts, and the like (Decker et al., 2023). It is also to be noted that clinicians may have to balance organizational mandates and client wishes pertaining to client identifiers in documentation.

When thinking about the specific language to use in clinical documentation, it is important that clinicians understand the historical context of terminology. One example of a term that has a deeply rooted historical context is "Hispanic" and "Latina/o," versus use of a specific country identifier, such as "Peruvian." Clinicians who ask direct questions get more accurate and robust information from the client.

It is also important to refer to one's professional ethical standards (beneficence, nonmaleficence, multicultural sensitivity) when considering which specific terms to use in documentation about clients. Furthermore, it is usually appropriate to discuss the preferred use of language in documentation with the client (Decker et al., 2023). This not only protects the client's autonomy but could also be incorporated into the informed consent.

Use of clear language is also imperative in protecting the clinician. Clear and timely clinical documentation can reduce the reliance on memory or memory error (Falvey et al., 2005; Zhang & Parsons, 2016). As mentioned earlier, there are times when the clinician's documentation is the only evidence of defense for a clinician who may be investigated for any ethical or legal reasons (HPSO, 2019). Outside the use of explicit, truthful, and objective language, it is also important that documentation be legible and easy to reference (Erford, 2015).

DOCUMENTATION FOR INSURANCE PURPOSES

Counseling, like any profession, depends on financial exchange, and monetary compensation can drive professional performance and outcomes. Mental health providers, like those in other professions, need to be monetarily compensated to provide and continue services. Compensation for mental health services rendered can be provided in several forms: self-pay, private insurance, state or federal programs, or grants, with third-party payers being the most frequent form of reimbursement (Sperry, 2005).

The Substance Abuse and Mental Health Services Administration (2021) reported that in 2020, only 10% of the mental services accessed were reimbursed through private health insurance, while 9% used Medicare, 11% used Medicaid, and 59% of other types of reimbursement were from a variety of other federal, state, and grant funds. According to the report, 89% of these were reimbursed with some form of third-party payer. The other 11% of the clients seen for mental health services were self-pay clients. These 11% of self-pay clients undoubtedly included some people who have private health insurance who chose not to use their insurance and provide self-pay for mental health services (Reif et al., 2012). Other clients who do not have health insurance would need to self-pay for mental health services.

Since third-party payers are the predominant source of payment for mental health services, clinicians may have extra challenges to overcome in providing services. One of these necessary tasks is to accurately and thoroughly document the basis for and execution of services provided (ACA, 2014; APA, 2017; NASW, 2021; Gutheil & Hilliard, 2001). Clinical documentation should be complete, objective, current, and timely in submission (HPSO, 2019). In addition, when a third-party payer is involved, clinical professionals are routinely required to provide a mental health diagnosis, as well as different levels of required clinical documentation, based on the third-party payer's guidelines and policies.

Facets of managed care in the framework of health care have been around for almost a century (Fox & Kongstvedt, 2013). Throughout the 1970s, the Health Maintenance Organization Act of 1973 started the allocation of federal funds for the expansion of service alternatives to the traditional forms of health care delivery and nonprofit managed care health insurance systems (Sanchez & Turner, 2003), which have become more involved in managing medical care. One of the key goals of managed care is to "decrease costs incurred by health insurance companies by eliminating waste and ensuring efficiency" (Gasquoine, 2010, p. 319). Since the induction of managed care in mental health treatment, there has been an emphasis on short-term psychotherapeutic approaches, with outcome assessment focused upon symptom reduction and functional improvement (Cantor & Fuentes, 2008; Sanchez & Turner, 2003). The emphasis on short-term services has increased, and managed care providers may require preauthorization of services; they can also determine the requirements for services and regulate the length of service, which can create an artificial termination of services (Gasquoine, 2010). These terms and procedures are individualized for the person in service and vary from third-party payer to third-party payer.

Whether the client is using private insurance, state or federal reimbursement, monetary allocations from a grant, or paying privately for services, the documentation of clinical services is essential in protecting the clinician and demonstrating valid care of the client (Gutheil & Hilliard, 2001). No matter the payment method, it is imperative that payment arrangements are not only discussed with the client but there is also a written agreement. If the client wants to use a third-party payer for services, then the client must provide written authorization for the clinician to bill the third-party payer (Barnett et al., 2014). Best practices for the method of payment agreement include the signed and dated original document being placed in the client's file with a copy provided to the client.

KEEPING, TRANSFERRING, RETAINING, AND DESTROYING CLINICAL DOCUMENTATION

During and after the therapeutic relationship, the client's records are to be protected (ACA, 2014; APA, 2017; NASW, 2021). The depth of detail related to these specifications varies per professional organization. However, each national organization addresses the retention, transferring, and destruction of client records.

Records Retention

Collectively, the *2014 ACA Code of Ethics* (ACA, 2014), the *Code of Ethics of the National Association of Social Workers* (NASW, 2021), and *Ethical Principles of Psychologists and Code of Conduct* (APA, 2017) direct clinicians to have suitable arrangements to retain client records in a secure location that prohibits unauthorized users from accessing the confidential client records. These guidelines protect the confidentiality of clients and recognize the client's records as protected health information that belongs to the client (Office for Civil Rights, 2022).

Client records are considered ongoing while the client is active in treatment, and at some point, the established therapeutic engagement does end. Termination of the therapeutic relationship can appear in many forms, such as:

- The client completes treatment.
- Treatment is no longer beneficial to the client.
- The client becomes incarcerated and will require a new intake when released.
- The client chooses to terminate treatment.
- The client's mandated treatment time expires.
- The client needs a higher level of care or treatment from a different provider.
- The insurance expires and the client can no longer afford to attend services.
- The client or clinician moves.
- The clinician retires or leaves the place of service.
- The client or clinician passes away.

Both the *2014 ACA Code of Ethics* (ACA, 2014) and the *Code of Ethics of the National Association of Social Workers* (NASW, 2021) provide recommendations for retaining documentation after the therapeutic relationship is terminated. Each of these organizations implores the clinician to follow state and federal statutes and policies that guide the retention and disposal of client records. This means that each clinician needs to be familiar with federal laws, as well as the specific state of practice's laws regarding keeping client records safe, maintaining confidentiality, and the length of time required to keep client records after the termination of services, no matter how the termination occurred. The *Ethical Principles of Psychologists and Code of Conduct* (APA, 2017) only specifies that the clinician should have advanced plans to preserve the client's confidentiality in the event they are no longer the client's treatment provider.

Records/Data Transfer

No matter the medium (verbal, electronic, or paper) used to transfer records, the ethical codes of the ACA (2014), NASW (2021), and APA (2017) guide clinicians to safeguard the process of transferring confidential information. The ACA (2014) and NASW (2021) codes denote clinicians are to retrieve written authorization from a client to communicate or transfer their records to authorized third parties, including third-party payers. The information in the *APA* (2017) code is not as thorough, only addressing the need for these clinicians to plan ahead in the event records need to be transferred and to assess the risks and limits to privacy through electronic transmission of information.

Both the ACA (2014) and NASW (2021) codes caution clinicians, in certain instances, to limit the client's access to their records, or portions of their records. Clinicians are guided to provide the client access to only portions of their records in circumstances where there are justifiable reasons the client or others may be harmed. If this occurs, the clinician is advised to document the client's request for the records and the rationale for withholding some or all the client's records. If the client receives a portion or all of their records, a clinical is ethically bound to be available to the client to assist them in interpreting their records (ACA, 2014; NASW, 2021).

Records Destruction

Although the client records belong to the individual client, there are provisions in place for a clinician or place of therapeutic engagement to dispose of inactive client data. Both the ACA (2014) and the NASW (2021) note that the disposal of client records needs to be consistent with the relevant laws that govern records and the licensing laws. The *ACA* (2014) code explicitly states that clinicians also need to carefully consider special records that include data that may be needed for future reference, such as in cases stemming from treatment related to court proceedings, abuse of a person's deemed incapable of consent, suicide, or violence.

Lastly, the ACA (2014), NASW (2021), and APA (2017) codes are very clear that clinicians need to have a designated person who will be the custodian of client records upon leaving the practice, whether by choice, incapacity, termination, or death. If a clinician is employed by an agency, the policies of the agency often address the guardianship of client records for the clinician. If the clinician is their own employer, it is imperative that the clinician not only plan for a guardian of records but also clearly provide this information to the client. Conversely, if the client passes away, both the ACA (2014) and *NASW* (2021) codes stress the need to maintain client confidentiality that reflects any legal parameters and respects any preferences indicated by the client. Again, the *APA* (2017) code only specifies that the clinician should have advanced plans to preserve the client's confidentiality in the event they are no longer the client's treatment provider.

None of the predominant mental health professional organizations, ACA, NASW, or APA, indicate a length of time between client contact and care and the destruction of client clinical data/documentation. HPSO (2019) suggests the clinician look to and follow the time frame established by their state and the federal laws, their licensing statutes, and any indications from third-party agreements. Furthermore, if there are multiple indications regarding records from the aforementioned organizations, then the clinician should follow the most stringent guideline.

In many instances, a clinician may not have clear guidance about a time frame to retain records before considering destroying them. HPSO (2019) does offer suggested time frames: 7 years for adult clients, at least 10 years for clients who are utilizing reimbursement through Medicaid or other forms of federal assistance, and for child/adolescent clients the recommended time of record retention is until the minor reaches "age of majority plus three years" (HPSO, 2019, p. 3). Clinicians are guided to seek out guidance from a court of law or their licensing board prior to destroying records that may be associated with cases or clients where child/elder abuse or neglect has been involved—and if there has been a suicide, assault, or violence (HPSO, 2019).

CONCLUSION

Federal and state laws and ethical principles and their codes regarding clinical documentation are in place to protect the client. Clients benefit from a clinician documenting their therapeutic interactions in many ways: With thorough clinical documentation of services provided, clients can potentially have their services reimbursed by an external payor. Clients will also have an ongoing record of services provided and received. If clients were to return to the same provider or have their services transferred, they have a past record of therapeutic services. Thorough clinical documentation can also prevent the client from receiving duplication of services or services that have not proven useful.

Federal and state laws and ethical principles and codes about clinical documentation are also in place to protect clinicians. Clinicians need to report by documenting any and all client interactions as best practice and timely rendering of services. Thorough clinical documentation supports treatment teams who are providing a myriad of services to the client by having a record of provider interactions and services rendered and therefore avoiding duplication of services. The major mental health organizations guide clinicians to document all professional interactions with clients, from the first professional engagement through discharge (ACA, 2014; APA, 2017; NASW, 2021). Before commencing therapeutic interactions, documentation such as informed consent, HIPAA agreements, and any necessary releases of information needs to be obtained. Across the remainder of the therapeutic interaction and as treatment progresses, other necessary documentation will be crafted or obtained (Erford, 2015).

Before the reader moves on to the subsequent chapters, the authors want to offer reassurance. Since clinicians report client contact through documentation, along with ethical, legal, and third-party reimbursement requirements, there will be plenty of opportunity to practice how to complete succinct clinical documentation through repetition. Do not fret or unduly struggle; oftentimes, mastery in succinctly documenting client data and interactions is developed through acquired clinical knowledge, repetition, and practice (Kodweis et al., 2021; Prieto & Scheel, 2002).

REFERENCES

American Counseling Association. (2014). *2014 ACA code of ethics.* https://www.counseling.org/docs/default-source/default-document-library/ethics/2014-aca-code-of-ethics.pdf

American Psychological Association. (2017). *Ethical principles of psychologists and code of conduct.* https://www.apa.org/ethics/code

Baird, B. (2005). *The Internship, practicum and field placement handbook: A guide for the helping professions (4th ed.).* Routledge.

Barnett, J., Zimmerman, J., & Walfish, S. (2014). *The ethics of private practice: A practical guide for mental health clinicians* (1st ed.). Oxford University Press.

Bertolote, J. M. (2008). Mental health policy paper: The roots of the concept of mental health. *World Psychiatry, 7,* 113–116.

Cantor, D. W., & Fuentes, M. A. (2008). Psychology's response to managed care. *Professional Psychology: Research and Practice, 39,* 638–645.

Decker, S. E., Farook, M. W., Meshberg-Cohen, S., Matsuura, T., Manning, M., Abel, E. A., Blakley, L., & Prelli, F. (2023). Clinical documentation of patient identities in the electronic health record: Ethical principles to consider. *Psychological Services.* Advance online publication. https://doi.org/10.1037/ser0000816

Erford, B. T. (2015). *Clinical experiences in counseling.* Pearson.

Falvey, J. E., Bray, T. E., & Hebert, D. J. (2005). Case conceptualization and treatment planning: Investigation of problem-solving and clinical judgment. *Journal of Mental Health Counseling, 27*(4), 348–372.

Fox, P. D., & Kongstvedt, P. R. (2013). A history of managed health care and health insurance in the United States. In P. D. Fox & P. R. Kongstvedt (Eds.), *The essentials of managed health care* (6th ed., pp. 1–36). Jones & Bartlett Learning.

Gasquoine, P. G. (2010). Comparison of public/private health care insurance parameters for independent psychological practice. *Professional Psychology: Research and Practice, 41*(4), 319–324.

Gutheil, T., & Hilliard, J. (2001). Don't write me down: Legal, clinical, and risk-management aspects of patients' requests that therapists not keep notes or records. *American Journal of Psychotherapy, 55,* 157–165.

Health Insurance Portability and Accountability Act, Pub. L. No. 104-191 (1996).

Health Providers Service Organization. (2019, March). *Counselor spotlight: Documentation excerpt from Counselor Liability Claim Report (2nd ed.).* https://www.hpso.com/Resources/Legal-and-Ethical-Issues/counselor-claim-report-second-edition

Health Providers Service Organization. (2021). *Counseling board complaint case study: Unprofessional conduct while providing services through a mental health therapy app.* https://www.hpso.com/Resources/Legal-and-Ethical-Issues/Counselor-Case-Study-Mental-Health-Therapy-App

Ivey, A. E., Ivey, M. B., & Zalaquett, C. P. (2018). *Intentional interviewing and counseling: Facilitating client development in a multicultural society.* (9th Ed.). Cengage Learning, Inc.

Kodweis, K., Schimmelfing, L. C., Yang, Y., & Persky, A. M. (2021). Methods for optimizing student pharmacist learning of clinical note writing. *American Journal of Pharmaceutical Education, 85*(2), 144–151.

Lorkowski, J., & Pokorski, M. (2022). Medical records: A historical narrative. *Biomedicines, 10*(2594), 1–13. https://doi.org/10.3390/biomedicines10102594

Modifications to the HIPAA Privacy, Security, Enforcement, and Breach Notification Rules, 45 C.F.R. § 160 & 164 (2013).

National Association of Social Workers. (2021). *Code of ethics of the National Association of Social Workers.* https://www.socialworkers.org/About/Ethics/Code-of-Ethics/Code-of-Ethics

Office for Civil Rights. (2022, October 19). *Summary of the HIPAA Privacy Rule.* U.S. Department of Health and Human Services. https://www.hhs.gov/hipaa/for-professionals/privacy/laws-regulations/index.html

Piazza, N. J., & Baruth, N. E. (1990). Client record guidelines. *Journal of Counseling & Development, 68,* 313–316.

Prieto, L. R., & Scheel, K. R. (2002). Using case documentation to strengthen trainees' case conceptualization skill. *Journal of Counseling & Development, 80,* 11–21.

Reif, S., Torres, M. E., Horgan. C. M., & Merrick, E. L. (2012). Characteristics of practitioners in a private managed behavioral health plan. *BMC Health Services Research, 12*(283), 1–6. https://doi.org/10.1186/1472-6963-12-283

Sanchez, L. M., & Turner, S. M. (2003). Practicing psychology in the era of managed care. *American Psychologist, 58*(2), 116–129.

Sheperis, C. J., Young, J. S., & Daniels, M. H. (2017). *Counseling Research: Quantitative, Qualitative, and Mixed Methods* (2nd Ed.). Pearson.

Sperry, L. (2005). Case conceptualization: A strategy for incorporating individual, couple, and family dynamics in the treatment process. *The American Journal of Family Therapy, 33,* 189–194.

Sperry, L. (2022). Adlerian case conceptualization and therapy: The pattern-focused approach. *The Journal of Individual Psychology, 78*(4), 465–478.

Substance Abuse and Mental Health Services Administration (2021). *2020 National Mental Health Services Survey (N-MHSS) annual report.* https://www.samhsa.gov/data/report/national-mental-health-services-survey-n-mhss-2020-data-mental-health-treatment-facilities

U.S. Department of Health and Human Services. (2022, October 20). *Individuals' right under HIPAA to access their health information.* https://www.hhs.gov/hipaa/for-professionals/privacy/guidance/access/index.html

Whiston, S. C. (2017). *Principles and applications of assessment in counseling.* (5th Ed.). Cengage Learning, Inc.

Zhang, N., & Parsons, R. D. (2016). *Field experience: Transitioning from student to professional.* Sage. https://doi.org/10.4135/9781483398709

CHAPTER 2

Clinical Case Vignettes

Gregory L. Bohner, PhD, and Daniel R. Romero, PhD

Case studies are beneficial as practice for mental health clinicians. Most of the chapters in this book utilize the two case studies below to illustrate how the reader can document client data in the clinical documentation. You are encouraged to refer to this chapter for review and application of the client's clinical data.

INTRODUCTION

Throughout the course of this book, there will be case examples utilized to demonstrate the application of client content to each of the documents discussed in the specific chapter. Two detailed cases will be used to show the progression of work with a client and the utilization of specific forms throughout treatment. The first case will be *The Case of Abel*, a story of a man in his 30s who is struggling with marital issues. Abel's case will be analyzed from a cognitive-behavioral theoretical perspective when appropriate. The second case will be *The Case of Susan*, a single mother in her 40s who recently lost her husband to a drug overdose and has made some significant life changes. Susan's case will utilize a reality therapy theoretical approach.

When reviewing any of the provided case studies, it is important to remember that case studies are inherently inflexible and incomplete in the assessment process. However, the goal is to provide some starting points for the reader to consider when they first begin to utilize clinical documentation. The full content of each case is included at the end of this chapter.

THE CASE OF ABEL

Abel is a 32-year-old male Ethiopian immigrant who resides in California. He is married to a Caucasian woman and together they have one male child, age 10. Abel is a truckdriver and is in school pursuing an associate's degree in accounting. Abel presents with periods of hopelessness, lethargy, and periodic suicidal thoughts. He describes his relationship with his wife as contentious.

Initial Assessment

Abel, a 32-year-old male, comes to the intake session of counseling because he is "unhappy with how things are going in his marriage" and he cannot "figure out how to make things work." When Abel came to see you for the first session, he smiled and shook your hand and asked, "How does this work?" He was restless and had a difficult time keeping his focus on the questions at hand. He reports that his wife, Mary, a 37-year-old White woman, does not listen to him and does not respect him. She constantly berates him, particularly in front of their 10-year-old son, Simon, and listens to her friends and family more than she listens to him. He is currently working as a truck driver in a local factory and is attending night classes to finish his associate's degree in accounting. His wife works as a hospital administrator. She is the primary breadwinner and provides them with a comfortable life, though they often argue about money. He also grew up in the Ethiopian Orthodox Tewahedo Church and wants Simon to attend church with him, while Mary grew up in a Reform Judaism synagogue and wants Simon to choose for himself.

Abel has told you that he is close to his mother, who has always been supportive of him, but has a tense relationship with his father. He was born in Ethiopia, but his family immigrated to Los Angeles when he was a teenager. He says that his father would berate him and call him "worthless." He says this is why he does not feel good about his work and does not think he can do anything to make people happy. He stopped caring about school until he got in trouble for egging his teacher's house in 10th grade. His family still lives in California, but his mother-in-law lives about 30 minutes away. She has never turned him away, but he thinks she was never happy that he married into the family, possibly because of his ethnicity. His father-in-law passed away 4 years ago.

Abel said that he will do well for a while, but every 9–12 months, he goes into a "funk." He does not like his work and just wants to sit in front of the TV all day long. He says this is when he gets into verbal fights with his wife, and these will sometimes turn physical (e.g., throwing pillows, punching walls, breaking decorations). Abel says his wife can "dish it out" as well as he can. According to Abel, he is a passionate person, and his wife is cold and emotionless until they fight. These funks last for about a month and then he starts to feel better again. They originally started about 10 years ago, but he feels like they have gotten worse over the past few years because he has started having thoughts of killing himself. He said these are usually in the form of thinking that everyone would be better off if he was not around. As you discussed these thoughts further, he denied any hallucinations and did not exhibit any delusional thinking.

When asked about his physical health, Abel says he has never had any major surgeries and regularly does his annual physical. He exercises three to four times a week, though this decreases during a funk. Abel stated that he is classified as overweight but says that is because he eats out for lunch every day. He came from work, and his clothes were neat and clean.

According to Abel, when he told his wife 6 months ago that he had been having suicidal thoughts for the past couple of years, she told him to do whatever he likes. He started to seriously contemplate killing himself, so he checked himself into a treatment hospital. When asked about how he would do so, he shrugs and says, "Probably drive somewhere so my son doesn't see me." He stayed at the hospital for 2 weeks and participated in group sessions and individual discussions about his life goals. As you continue to talk with Abel, he acknowledges who he is and can identify the current year and where you are meeting.

Abel is seeing you as follow-up treatment and to continue working on making his marriage and life "more bearable." He wants to figure out how to better communicate with his wife and take control of his thoughts for his little boy. He says that he has been feeling good lately, with no thoughts of suicide, and definitely doesn't want to hurt anyone else but wouldn't be surprised if a funk started soon. "I just really want to get on top of this so it doesn't become a bigger issue."

Session #3

Abel comes to see you for his third session. He has rescheduled the past 2 weeks because of sickness. As Abel walks into the session, his eyes are downcast, and his nose is red. He apologizes for missing the past 2 weeks and thanks you for meeting with him. He shares that in the past couple of weeks, the fighting between him and his wife has intensified. The other night, Simon mentioned going to dinner with Mary and her friend from work Marcus. Simon also said Mary was laughing and smiling throughout the meal and was "happier than she has been in a long time." Abel says he is not sure what he wants to do moving forward, but he cannot stop thinking that Mary is cheating on him and maybe he should just get a divorce. When you explore the topic further, Abel denies that he has had any suicidal ideation, but he does think this has led to him being in a funk again. When you ask about his behavior the past few weeks, Abel shares that he has been drinking more and eating poorly. However, he insists that he was diagnosed with the flu a week and a half ago and that is why he has canceled appointments. Abel reiterates that he thinks the sessions with you are important and that he is committed to doing better. As you finish the session, Abel decides that one of his goals is to eat more healthy meals for lunch. Instead of stopping at a fast food restaurant every day, he decides to make his lunch for 3 out of the 5 work days. He also decides to spend at least one night with just him and Simon because his son "is the most important thing in the world."

Session #6

This marks the fourth week in a row that Abel has come to therapy. He says that he is consistently taking his lunch 4 days a week and only eats out on the day he spends with some coworkers. He also has enjoyed bowling with Simon once a week in the father-son league at the local bowling alley.

At the present time, Abel wants to figure out how to confront Mary about the time she spends with Marcus. Abel thinks he has worked enough on himself and that Mary owes it to him to be honest about whether or not there is something else happening. As you reflect with him on his motivations for questioning Mary, Abel reveals that his father cheated on his mother when Abel was a teenager. Abel found out about the incident and threatened to reveal the truth to his mother. His father called him the equivalent of a "good-for-nothing, lazy ass." Unwilling for Simon to experience the same conflict, Abel says he must know the truth and whether it is time to end his marriage. You thank Abel for his honesty and the courage to be vulnerable in session. Abel agrees to do journal writing over the course of the next week to give himself time to reflect on how he wants to move forward in a way that is healthiest for himself, Mary, and Simon. He says the plan is to take time each morning before he drives his route to do the journaling.

Session #10

Abel has missed 3 out of the last 4 weeks of sessions. He calls the day before to reschedule for the next week at the same time. At the beginning of the current session, you reiterate the importance of working consistently in order to achieve Abel's goals of increasing his mental well-being and strengthening the relationship with his family. As a way of bolstering his work so far, you reflect on the progress he has made in exercising consistently, eating a healthier diet, and spending time with Simon. You ask whether the day and time are still the best fit for Abel's schedule. As you are talking, Abel appears to become more agitated. When you ask what his current thoughts are, Abel says therapy is obviously a waste of time. Angrily, he says, "All of the things you told me to do haven't changed anything!" He reveals that Mary still cheated on him with Marcus. It is only 15 minutes into the session, but Abel storms out. You call him later that day to discuss rescheduling so he can talk further about how he wants to move forward, but he does not return any of your phone calls or emails over the course of the next week. You complete his termination letter and add it to his client file. Finally, you schedule a reminder to call one more time a week later to attempt to reestablish a connection and provide an opportunity for further sessions or referrals to other therapists.

Session #11

It has been 3 months since you have heard from Abel. He arrives at your office one morning at opening, full of desperation, and says he needs to see you right away. You have an open appointment and ask Abel to give you 5 minutes to prepare your office. He sits in the waiting room, continuously wringing his hands and rubbing them on his pant legs. He is wearing sweatpants and a baggy T-shirt that is too large.

When Abel enters the office, he starts talking before you can completely close the door. He starts by apologizing for the way he left your office the last time and says he was "just so upset about everything." He relays to you that he recently moved out of his house and has begun divorce proceedings with Mary. As he was cleaning out some of his belongings this morning, he noticed a book under the dining room table. When he opened it up, he realized he was reading his son's journal. It fell to the last page where it was written, "I wish Dad would just man up and do what it takes to win Mom back. But he never finishes anything he starts, so I don't think that will happen." Abel tells you this has sent him into a spiral and he cannot stop thinking about killing himself. "If my own son cannot see me as a man, perhaps I should just get out of the way and let Marcus raise him. My dad was right all along; I'm just a waste of space."

As you discuss the situation further with Abel, he shares that he was about to go back to his new apartment and get the gun that he owns to shoot himself. He knows a field not far from his work where no one goes to, and it wouldn't make a fuss. But before reaching the apartment, he started worrying about whether or not he should go through with it and knew he had to contact you.

After Abel has an opportunity to share, you thank him for coming to your office and express your genuine desire to help him decide on the next steps moving forward. You also affirm how difficult it feels to face rejection from his son. After processing further, Abel agrees to completing a safety plan and wants to restart regular counseling sessions. Following the session, you reach out to Dr. Lin Son, a trusted colleague, and consult about the session. Dr. Son affirms your choice of action but recommends Abel revisit the treatment hospital that provided his initial services. He recommends you call Abel with this suggestion and document the day and time of the call as well as Abel's response.

THE CASE OF SUSAN

Susan Thomas is a 43-year-old single mother of three children under age 10. She is currently enrolled in a clinical mental health counseling program at a midsize Midwestern college. Susan's decision to pursue a counseling degree stemmed from a personal tragedy: Her husband passed away 3 years ago due to an accidental drug overdose. Motivated by this experience, Susan embarked on a path to become a substance abuse counselor, aiming to help others navigate similar challenges.

Presenting Problem

Susan has recently begun experiencing significant stress related to her coursework, specifically during exams and presentations. While she did well in her undergrad psychology program, it was so long ago, and Susan feels that she is not as knowledgeable and skilled with the technical aspects that are required. She often feels behind in her studies and she has to stay up late and work harder than other students in order to feel caught up. Susan feels like she has to spend all of her non-work time on schoolwork, which has become increasingly challenging both emotionally and academically. There are times when it becomes almost impossible to focus, especially when the readings and assignments make her feel that maybe there was more that she could have done to help her husband.

Susan also feels increasingly overwhelmed by the demands of balancing her responsibilities as a mother and a graduate student. Susan's anxiety has started affecting her sleep, appetite, and overall well-being, leading her to seek individual counseling support.

Initial Assessment

In the initial session, Susan shows up 10 minutes early and is eager to begin counseling. She is wearing wireless earbuds in the waiting room area and quickly removes them when she is called back for the interview. Susan is dressed in casual business attire and looks well-put-together and confident in her demeanor. She speaks to you very firmly and confidently, with a comfortable amount of eye contact, as you invite her into your office and ask about her day and what brings her into counseling. As she begins to share her story, Susan becomes visibly emotional when talking about her family, her voice shaking as she at first tries to hold back tears and then reaches for a tissue when they can no longer be contained. Susan apologizes to you for becoming emotional and says, "I told myself that I wouldn't do that here today; I was going to keep it together."

Susan shares current challenges in pursuing her counseling degree. She expresses feeling overwhelmed by academic stress, imposter syndrome, and the demands of parenthood. Susan's grief over her husband's death also emerges as a significant emotional burden. At one point she puts her hands together on her lap while closing her eyes and says in a soft voice, "I know that I should be moving beyond this, but being in this program seems to be bringing up unresolved issues that I thought I had worked through. I guess that's part of why I'm here."

Susan goes on to share that she was living in a small town and moved to a larger city in her state in order to be closer to family and resources for her children. While Susan indicates that she was never close to her mother, she thought that moving closer would strengthen their relationship and that her mother would be able to help out with childcare while Susan was busy with work and school. During the intake Susan also details current stressors, including lack of consistent childcare and feeling empty and alone. Susan expresses a strong desire to succeed in her counseling program but feels unsure about managing the academic workload; she has also begun to feel imposter syndrome, including thoughts of worthlessness. Though Susan often has thoughts of "Who am I to think that I can help anyone?" she also believes that she needs to "do this" in order to feel good about herself and tells herself, "I am doing this for you [her husband]."

Counseling Goals

Identified goals that you established with Susan:

1. Develop coping strategies to manage academic stress and anxiety effectively.
2. Improve time management and organizational skills to balance coursework and parenting responsibilities.
3. Address any unresolved grief or emotional challenges related to Susan's husband's death.
4. Enhance self-care practices to promote overall well-being and resilience.

Counseling Process

As Susan's counselor, you quickly establish a therapeutic rapport, including an empathic and collaborative approach with Susan. Together with Susan, you explore her coping mechanisms and identify triggers for her anxiety, such as use of technology, assignment and reading deadlines, exams, and feelings of inadequacy. You introduce relaxation techniques, mindfulness exercises, and stress management strategies tailored to Susan's needs.

Together, you and Susan create a realistic study schedule that accommodates Susan's parenting duties while allowing dedicated time for coursework. You work collaboratively on setting achievable goals, breaking tasks into manageable steps, and prioritizing self-care activities. Susan learns to challenge negative self-talk and perfectionistic tendencies, replacing them with self-compassion and a growth mindset.

In addition to academic support, you provide a safe space for Susan to process her grief and emotions surrounding her husband's death. Together, you explore coping strategies for managing triggers, fostering resilience, and finding meaning and purpose in Susan's journey as a counselor and a mother.

Session #4

Susan begins this session by expressing a larger than usual amount of self-doubt. As the session progresses, Susan shares that the anniversary of her husband's passing is approaching, and she is struggling: "This is all just too much for me. I don't think I can go on." You demonstrate warmth and concern for Susan, and she goes on to describe her past week, saying, "This is the worst I've felt in a long time," and "This is just not what I expected it would be." You go on to acknowledge and validate Susan's feelings and concerns and let her know that it is understandable that she is feeling this resurgence of emotions and grief, especially as the anniversary comes near. Together, you and Susan review treatment goals and decide to focus on the goals that would help Susan to feel supported and less overwhelmed. You remind Susan that for the past couple of sessions, she hasn't talked about her deceased husband and her feelings too much and instead has been very focused on talking about her schoolwork and the challenges of being a good mother while maintaining a good grade point average in the counseling program. Susan agrees that she sometimes tries to "just not think about things" and that it may be helpful for you to help her to identify and talk about her feelings more, even though it might be difficult, because "I know that nothing can bring him back, so I sometimes don't feel like talking about it is good for me." After spending the remainder of the session tearfully talking about her feelings of sadness and loneliness, Susan acknowledges that it might be important for her to acknowledge and express her feelings in counseling.

Session #8

Susan comes to the session with excitement that she passed all of her courses, even the one that she thought would be impossible to pass, saying, "I can't believe that I passed and did so well with all of my courses. I am so glad that I stuck with it. I feel so many emotions and feel like crying right now." You congratulate Susan for her accomplishments and allow her space to share her excitement. As Susan talks about her feelings of relief and happiness to be done with the semester, she suddenly starts to choke up and gets quiet. You suspect that Susan's abrupt quietness is because of her thinking about her deceased husband and grief. You give Susan space to be in her feelings and demonstrate empathy with your body language and face. You assure Susan that whatever it is she is feeling is okay to feel and talk about with you. Susan tears up and says, "I just wish that he was still here and that he could at least see what I am doing and know that I am doing this for him."

Session #12

This is Susan's final session. She arrives at the appointment 10 minutes early. As she walks in and situates herself in your office, you ask how her day is going and she smiles and says, "It's been great so far. I had an early morning workout at the gym this morning, so my head feels crisp and clear." Susan goes on to tell you that she has been making great progress on her workout and self-care goals and that her children have also noticed a change in her, saying that she seems more relaxed and confident.

The past three sessions have focused on Susan's needs and self-care. You have also worked with Susan on building her community network and connecting her with a women's community support group. Susan has learned that it will be important for her to pay attention to her self-care and wellness needs and that she may experience days when she feels discouraged and disconnected from herself and others. Susan is feeling much better, and you work with her to update the safety plan and plan for continued progress. Susan asks about checking in from time to time to review her progress, as she feels like working with you has been so helpful. You discuss with her how this may happen and let her know that she is always welcome to reach out if she if she needs to.

CONCLUSION

Now that you are familiar with the cases of Abel and Susan, you will have the opportunity to apply these cases to practice the different types of clinical documentation in the subsequent chapters.

CHAPTER 3

Informed Consent

Marisa L. White, PhD, Keeley Stewart, PhD, Mona Gallo, EdD, Darlene Vaughn, PhD, and Daniel R. Romero, PhD

INTRODUCTION

Informed consent is the cornerstone of the counseling process, making it the cornerstone of the documentation process. The informed consent form is likely one of the first documents that clients read, sign, and get a copy of, as it is needed before any services are provided to the client. It is important to note that informed consent is an ethical and legal mandate, and as a result, it must be documented correctly to protect the client, counselor, and other stakeholders.

Informed consent is defined in counseling as clients having the freedom of choice about either entering or remaining in a counseling relationship and being provided adequate information about the counseling process and the clinician (American Counseling Association [ACA], 2014; American Psychological Association [APA], 2017; National Association of Social Workers [NASW], 2021). Clinicians are directed to review, both in writing and verbally along with the client, the rights and responsibilities of both the clinician and client. Informed consent occurs throughout the counseling process, and clinicians will document discussions of informed consent throughout the counseling relationship (ACA, 2014; APA, 2017).

There are four components that must be considered when determining legal informed consent: "capacity, voluntariness, decision-making, and knowledge" (Dalal, 2020, p. 6). *Capacity* refers to a person's legal competence, whereas *decision-making* in this context is a medical term that refers to a person's ability to decide on their care. In short, to provide consent, a client must be of "sound mind" at the time of consent.

Voluntariness indicates a client must be acting of their own free will. Finally, the component of *knowledge* implies the client has enough information, including information about the nature and consequences of the treatment, to make an informed decision (Dalal, 2020).

Informed consent is a contract between a professional who provides a service or treatment and an individual/set of individuals (client or group) receiving the service or treatment. Informed consent is part of the research, clinical/counseling, supervision, consultation, and education processes. Many agencies prescribe what is included in the consent for each of these specialty areas.

INFORMED CONSENT IS UNIQUE

Documenting the informed consent process is different than other documentation for several reasons. As stated before, informed consent is a legal and ethical requirement. Another aspect that makes the informed consent document unique is that before allowing a client to sign a consent form, the clinician must determine their ability to legally and ethically consent. Factors that may impact one's ability to consent include age, mental capacity, treatment level, or legal limitations. One example is a 9-year-old child would be unable to consent to treatment even if they are the primary client. Another example is a person with diminished capacity who may not be able to legally sign an informed consent and may require permission from a legal guardian. Other special limitations would be a client's capacity to consent to treatment if the client is under the influence of a substance or if they have severe mental illness symptoms (e.g., psychosis or being in a catatonic state).

Another way informed consent is different from other clinical documentation is that this document is reviewed by the client. But informed consent is not just a document; it is also a process that clinicians must document in other clinical documentation throughout the length of treatment. A client needs to read and sign an informed consent form before the start of treatment. The process of verbally reviewing the informed consent form in the initial meeting should also be documented in a case note. Consent should be revisited numerous times throughout the treatment process. For example, a clinician may discuss the concept of informed consent with a client who has been in treatment for 3 months because that client would like to access their records. If the consent contained information about how to obtain the records, this information would be reviewed. A clinician may also discuss consent with a client who has disclosed information that must be reported to officials. When a clinician must report suspected child or elder abuse, it is likely that this breach of confidentiality is discussed with the client. Discussing the limitations of confidentiality is a return to the informed consent form.

When consent is reviewed in session, that discussion should be documented in a case note. Consequently, informed consent is more than just a document with a client's or proxy's signature.

The final unique factor about the informed consent document is that it is one of the documents that is reviewed with the client in writing and verbally (ACA, 2014; NASW, 2021). This is not the case for documents like case notes, termination summaries, or other documents that are part of mental health treatment. Additional information about working with clients who cannot consent due to limitations in capacity or decision-making will be discussed later in this chapter.

ETHICAL NEED FOR INFORMED CONSENT

As identified, all the predominant mental health organizations' codes of ethics are clear that clients are to receive informed consent for service (ACA, 2014; APA, 2017; NASW, 2021). Although it is presumed that the process of informed consent would be in writing, it is only clearly defined in the *2014 ACA Code of Ethics* (ACA, 2014) and the *Ethical Principles of Psychologists and Code of Conduct* (APA, 2017). And although the *Code of Ethics of the National Association of Social Workers* (NASW, 2021) provides clear guidance to clinicians obtaining informed consent, it does not specifically delineate the need for informed consent to be in writing.

Outside of written informed consent, the ACA's (2014) code denotes that counselors are obligated to provide informed consent verbally and that the process is ongoing throughout the treatment process. The APA (2017) code also recognizes there can be verbal consent and explicitly notes that whether written or verbal, the client's consent or permission needs to be documented in writing. Although not clearly noted in the NASW's (2021) code, it is implied that informed consent is verbal, but it is not explicitly noted that the informed consent process is ongoing.

The *2014 ACA Code of Ethics* (ACA, 2014) provides what seems like an exhaustive list of items to include within the informed consent process, including purposes, goals, risks, benefits, procedures, techniques, approaches, client engagement, changes in modality, continuation, limits, refusal, and any consequences of the refusal of treatment. Included in this list is appropriate disclosure of the clinician's credentials, experience, and any qualifications. Implications of a diagnosis, testing, and reporting are to be explicitly explained to clients, as well as any intended uses of the above. Payment procedures, billing and lack of payment procedures, as well as access to records are also noted. The code is very clear that the right to confidentiality belongs to the client; however, the clinician is delegated to clearly explain any and all limitations. Because the informed consent for clinicians affiliated with the ACA is ongoing, clients are provided with the opportunity of ongoing consent for treatment and can choose to engage in, continue with, or terminate treatment with the clinician (ACA, 2014).

The *Ethical Principles of Psychologists and Code of Conduct* (APA, 2017) notes that the informed consent process needs to be addressed as early as possible, implying some clients may not be able to initially consent. It is clearly outlined that clinicians are to inform clients about the fees, any third-party involvement, any limits of confidentiality, potential risks, available alternative treatment, as well as the essence and potential direction of therapy. In addition, clinicians must present any limits of confidentiality in the informed consent, indicate that a client's participation in treatment is voluntary, and provide the client with adequate opportunity to ask questions and obtain answers (APA, 2017).

The *Code of Ethics of the National Association of Social Workers* (NASW, 2021) recognizes that the language used during the informed consent process should be clear and presented in a manner where the client can understand the explanation of the purpose, risks, limits, costs, and alternatives of services, as well as the client's ultimate decision to refuse or withdraw consent. These clinicians are also ethically required to provide a time frame of the consent while allowing the clients to ask questions (NASW, 2021).

INABILITY TO PROVIDE CONSENT AND MANDATED CLIENTS

Although this chapter started by stating that consent is the cornerstone of the counseling process, there are limitations to informed consent. These limitations typically involve minors and adults who are legally incapacitated. It is important to acknowledge that there are exceptions to the exceptions. Typically, minors cannot provide legal consent. This is not always the case when it comes to consenting to mental health or addiction treatment. State laws dictate the age of consent for mental health and addiction treatment for individuals. For example, Maryland's age of consent for mental health treatment is 12 years old, whereas Texas's is 18 years old (World Population Review, 2024). States also dictate who can take away consent. For example, in Maine, a minor child 14 years or older can consent to their own treatment for substance use or mental health without parental/guardian acknowledgment or revocation, and if the parent/guardian consents for the minor's treatment, the minor may not revoke it (An Act to Define the Age of Consent for Alcohol or Drug Treatment and Mental Health Services, 1995).

Some states also limit how many sessions a client can receive before informing their legal guardian. States may decide who can consent based on the level of treatment. For example, Ohio requires legal guardian consent for inpatient treatment; but a client who is 14 years old can consent for outpatient treatment. In Connecticut, minors can only consent to six sessions before the clinician requires guardian consent (World Population Review, 2024). These details are important for counselors in the consent process, as laws inform the information included in the consent and who can ethically and legally sign such documentation and provide consent to treatment.

It is also important to note that age of consent being related to a numerical age is a concept that is uniquely Western. Many cultures distinguish maturity and decision-making ability based on other factors. In some Asian cultures, for instance, moral maturity is determined by a person's ability to understand the connection and balance between the community and the individual (Ekmekci & Arda, 2017). In addition, legal age does not necessarily indicate relational autonomy in all families or cultures. As a result, mental health professionals must be aware of how consent is conceptualized in different cultures and adjust accordingly (see the Culturally Relevant Informed Consent section later in this chapter).

Guardianship or Conservatorship

Determining who can provide consent may not be clear-cut. Mental health professionals must be aware of how their state determines who can make decisions on an individual's behalf. It is important to understand the terms "legal guardian" and "conservator," as they are terms to describe individuals who can consent for a client. These terms may have different definitions based on location, and it is the clinician's responsibility to understand the terms' meaning in their state(s) of practice. Typically, *guardianship* refers to a person who helps with day-to-day decision-making for individuals, whereas *conservatorship* is often used when a person (authority) helps an individual with financial decisions. Mental health treatment consent often pertains to both day-to-day decision-making and finances (e.g., cost of treatment, access to insurance, etc.), and as a result, mental health professionals may have contact with a guardian or conservator.

Even when guardianship or custody seems more straightforward, it is always recommended the clinician ask if the person has the legal ability to consent for the client. In reality, the client may live with someone who they call a parent or relative and state that they have custody, but that may not be the case legally. For example, a minor may be raised by a grandparent, but the legal paperwork was never filed to give the grandparent legal guardianship. In addition, a client may also be transported to sessions by a person who is not legally allowed to consent to treatment; thus, the issue of consent may need to be discussed prior to the first meeting (possibly during the phone intake or appointment scheduling process). In these cases, it is customary to ask the client or guardian to provide documentation of guardianship or to sign a statement indicating that they can consent for the mental health treatment of the client.

Divorce

In situations of divorce, consent for treatment of a custodial person can become complicated, to say the least. It is recommended that the client bring proof of the divorce decree that indicates who can provide consent to treatment. If the divorce documents do not indicate the decision-making ability of the individual parents (as it relates to mental health treatment), it is ideal that both parents consent to treatment. In circumstances where both parents are not present to consent or the documents are not being provided, a clinician may want the presenting parent to sign a statement indicating that they have the legal right to sign consent for treatment without the consent of the alternate parent. This would be an additional consent form to include in the client's clinical file. It is also important to note that each state may have laws about who is the legal guardian and who could consent to the client's treatment if the parents never married. Some states automatically grant primary custody to the mother, whereas others provide joint custody. Clinicians who work with minors will want to be aware of unmarried custody laws in their state of practice and speak to their agency and/or supervisor about what additional documentation is needed for consent in specific cases.

It is important to note that a stepparent cannot typically consent to treatment. Yes, a stepparent may be a primary caretaker and engaged as the "parent" of the client, but they do not have the same legal rights as the biological parent unless they are designated as a legal guardian or adoptive parent.

Informed Assent

When counseling a minor, an adult who is legally incapacitated, or other people unable to give voluntary consent, clinicians may seek the assent of the client and still include them in the decision-making processes. Consent is a legal agreement, whereas *assent* is an aspirational concept and may be used to build trust and rapport with clients. Despite not being required by many mental health organizations, the National Association of School Psychologists (2020) does recommend the use of assent. Alternatively, the APA (2017) provides specific guidance for obtaining assent: Clinicians are guided to deliver a suitable explanation while seeking the client's assent. Clinicians consider the benefits for the client, as well as their preferences.

Like informed consent, informed assent can be a document kept in the client's file and may be mentioned in other documentation. Assent forms typically look similar to informed consent and include the risks and benefits of treatment; however, it is adapted according to the client's age and comprehension level. It is important to note that assent does not replace informed consent. Informed consent is required (where legally applicable), and assent is an extra document and process that may be used to provide a sense of dignity and autonomy to a client who is not able or allowed to provide informed consent.

Mandated Clients

Clients who are mandated or court-ordered to attend treatment go through the same informed consent procedures as other clients. What makes these clients a unique population is that they are often mandated by an official body (authority) that will require them to enter treatment and release information about their engagement in treatment to an agency or official. Being "mandated" often makes clients feel like they do not have a choice to or not to consent and that they are not voluntarily entering into treatment. Despite feeling that treatment is not voluntary, mandated clients can choose to not consent to treatment. In actuality, the client is choosing to enter treatment to meet some qualification set by the court or authority. Treatment may be a step the client takes to earn custody of their children, provided as an alternative to jail, or a condition of probation/parole. In these cases, mandated clients are technically agreeing to treatment to meet the requirement of the authority. Mandated clients can also choose not to consent or obtain treatment and accept the consequences of that choice. The same would be true for a client who enters treatment because their partner used treatment as an ultimatum. They are not mandated to receive treatment, but they may attend counseling because they do not want to endure the consequences of not attending treatment.

Outside of the benefits of counseling, there can be risks for a client. For example, clients may experience discomfort when discussing painful and difficult situations, counseling may be challenging, and treatment may not be effective for everyone. In the case of clients who are mandated to treatment, confidentiality may be limited. A mandated client's information could be used by the mandating institution in ways that may not be beneficial to the client. An example might be if the client reveals that they have relapsed, using an illegal substance, then that information could be shared with the court and the probation officer could decide that the client has violated their probation and needs to be reproved.

Another risk for mandated clients is that information will be reported to the overseeing agency (mandator). It is advisable for the clinician and client to discuss what information will be documented from each treatment engagement and how that information will be shared with the overseeing agency (mandator). For example, will case notes be shared or just the dates of attendance? If the cases notes are shared, the clinician may want to also discuss what kind of information is included in the case notes.

Another risk when working with mandated clients is the client's choice to miss treatment and/or prematurely terminate treatment outside of the mandated length of time. Although clinicians want to support a client's ability to make autonomous choices, they also need to be clear with mandated clients about any potential consequences for missing treatment or terminating services outside the mandated treatment time frame. Ensuring that the client understands the risks related to mandated treatment is essential so that the client can determine if they want to consent to the conditions of treatment. Clinicians need to document these discussions related to missing treatment and premature termination of services and the potential consequences regarding both. Confirming that the client understands the risks associated with the information being released to the mandating agency and any consequences of missed treatment or premature termination is ensuring beneficence and nonmaleficence.

CRITICAL CONTENT FOR INFORMED CONSENT DOCUMENTATION

When developing an informed consent, some clinicians may choose to use examples found on the internet. This may be appropriate to use as a checks-and-balances system after one creates the informed consent form, but it may not be sufficient in creating a complete or appropriate informed consent document. It is also important to note that clinicians should routinely assess the quality and accuracy of the informed consent document. Again, this is not just a document that is completed at intake and archived; it is the entire process that is documented.

The content included in an informed consent document will differ depending on a variety of factors. Many clinicians have multiple informed consent documents that are tailored to a client population (e.g., minors, couples, groups, mandated, etc.) or the method of counseling provided. It is recommended that clinicians have an informed consent document for telehealth counseling and a different document for in-person mental health services. Some clinicians have separate informed consent documents for counseling with minors, groups, families, couples, and individuals. It is important to note that when a clinician has more than one client in a session, all clients must provide consent for treatment.

Professional factors may also influence what a clinician includes in or excludes from an informed consent. Before creating the informed consent document, a clinician should consider what is required and recommended by insurance providers, state laws, licensure boards, certification-granting agencies, professional organizations, codes of ethics, and best practice guidelines for the specific profession, area of practice, and specialty area of expertise. Some clinicians may need to consider complementary and conflicting recommendations based on their credentials. This may occur for clinicians who are licensed in multiple states or hold different licensures (e.g., Licensed Social Worker and Licensed Professional Counselor).

When creating or updating an informed consent document, the clinician must use their clinical judgment to determine the level of detail provided in the document. This will likely differ depending on the agency, clinician, client population being served, cultural norms, or changes in ethical codes and laws. The level of detail to provide in the informed consent may also vary due to ethical requirements. For example, the *2014 ACA Code of Ethics* (ACA, 2014) states that clinicians need to provide adequate information about the counseling process, as well as the clinician. It is up to the individual clinician to determine what constitutes "adequate information." Interestingly, the *Ethical Principles of Psychologists and Code of Conduct* (APA, 2017) and the *Code of Ethics of the National Association of Social Workers* (NASW, 2021) do not indicate that a clinician must provide information about the clinician in the informed consent; thus, what to include is up to the individual clinician. It is important to find a balance between too much and too little detail. Clinicians may be tempted to provide more detail as a protective measure, but it is important to remember that too much information could overwhelm the client and contribute to them not reading the consent. Cultural considerations should also inform the informed consent process. For example, many "Muslim client do not expect or desire a great deal of explicit information. Paradoxically, too much information can leave them to feel uninformed and can even generate distrust" (Tham et al., 2022, p. 7). This emphasizes the importance of balance. Clinicians must provide the client with enough details so they are better able to make an informed decision about treatment, but they also do not want to flood the client with miniscule details that will deter the client from truly consenting to treatment.

As noted previously, informed consent is not a static document but an ongoing process that will require updating. A good example of the need to update informed consent processes documents occurred during COVID-19 pandemic. At this time, adjustments were made to clinical practice; thus, the informed consent forms and processes needed to be updated to add information about telehealth, safety risks and requirements, and attendance. Updating informed consent also needs to occur if a law or ethical code has changed and has adjusted clinical treatment. This occurred in 2022 when the No Surprise Act was put into effect (APA, 2021). At this time, clinicians were required to inform clients of the expected charges for treatment. If a client was already in treatment, this act required that clinicians add an addendum to the consent (APA, 2021). Additional reasons to update an informed consent or add an addendum to the informed consent would be if the client turned 18, the counselor changed the type of treatment offered, a change in technology platform used, a change in pay structure or collection procedures, and so on.

CULTURALLY RELEVANT INFORMED CONSENT

Consent must be more than a procedural or legal process. Special consideration for culture must be given in all areas of clinical practice and documentation. This is particularly important in mental health treatment and with informed consent. Autonomy (voluntariness) is the basis of informed consent, yet it is a value not shared by all cultures. In some intercultural groups, "communities prioritize the consent of community leaders or the head of the family" over consent of the individual (Ekmekci & Arda, 2017, p. 159). Personhood is a concept of individualism in Western cultures, whereas non-Western cultures are only realized through connection and community (Ekmekci & Arda, 2017). As a result, mental health clinicians must contemplate how to respect a non-Western client's cultural values (of interdependence and communal decision-making) as well as the Western ethical codes and laws that require consent based on individual autonomy.

The importance of cultural competence can be reflected in documentation, including informed consent. The clinician must consider how the effects of a client's culture may impact the informed consent process, and the clinician should alter their practices where applicable (ACA, 2014; NASW, 2021). An example of making the informed consent culturally relevant is to explain that although the ethical code focuses on the Western notion of individual autonomy, the clinician can also work with the family or community stakeholders, when culturally relevant, once the release-of-information form is completed.

Clinicians should also consider how cultural relativism is related to language and how language is understood within culture. When creating an informed consent document, it is important to consider if the information is available in the client's primary language, free from professional jargon, and appropriate for the client's reading and comprehension level. Clinicians may consider consulting with cultural experts and asking them to review their informed consent document to understand the cultural implications that the document or process may have with clients from certain cultures.

Special attention should be paid when obtaining informed consent from marginalized populations. Historically, clinicians and researchers have misused informed consent processes to take advantage of, hurt, and kill marginalized populations. For more information on this topic, research the Tuskegee Study, the eugenics movement, or American Indian "boarding schools." Acknowledging the historical deceit and allowing space for questions and alternative explanations is one step that clinicians can take to increase trust during the informed consent process.

Mental health clinicians must communicate information in a manner that is developmentally and culturally appropriate for the specific client. Clinicians are expected to use clear language that the client can understand from their cultural context/worldview. If the client has difficulty understanding the language, the clinician is responsible for providing an informed consent document that the client can comprehend (ACA, 2014; APA, 2017; NASW, 2021). There are several ways to cross-culturally improve the informed consent process: Clinicians can allow the client to take information home or have a friend or family member present, provide a video about consent, use pictures to illustrate key ideas, provide a summary, use large print, and provide sufficient time for questions and answers (Quinn et al., 2013).

INFORMATION NEEDED IN THE INFORMED CONSENT

The informed consent agreement between the clinician and the client establishes the expectations for each member of the therapeutic relationship. It is important for the informed consent document to be professional, ethical, and appropriate for the client's level of understanding. Consent forms need to be thorough and easy to understand. Informed consent is crucial for communication of how the counseling relationship works and allows for the disclosure of legal limitations and compliance. Again, this important piece of clinical documentation includes the responsibilities of the clinician, as well as the expectations of the client. The informed consent document should contain important business policies and the anticipated delivery of services, as well as the disclosure of risks and benefits of therapy. Ultimately, the informed consent document assists in the empowerment of the client, encouraging collaboration and a sound therapeutic alliance between the clinician and the client, and creates a baseline for ethical principles and judgment.

A thorough and specific informed consent should provide the client with the understanding that the services they are about to receive are protected by a contract. Each member of the counseling relationship has their own responsibilities to fulfill. In the initial meeting of the clinician and the client, details of the informed consent must be discussed, and the questions answered. The beginning of the counseling relationship is important and must not be hurried.

When composing a new informed consent document, careful attention is given to every aspect of the business as well as the counseling relationship. This document must include many items but, in sum, must include these major elements: disclosure of information; competency of the client (or the surrogate) and legalities therein; the ethical obligations of the clinician; and nature and progress of the counseling relationship.

Critical Items to Include

There are many critical items to include on the informed consent form that can assist the client in understanding their rights and gain clarity of the counseling process. The data included may also aid in protecting the clinician.

Benefits of Participating in Counseling

The client will likely benefit greatly from what they learn while in counseling. Counseling can provide the client with a better understanding of themselves and the way they perceive situations, better coping skills, a higher sense of self-worth, and better communication strategies. Open interactions from the counselor can assist the client.

Risks of Engaging in Counseling

Some clients may experience unexpected and unwelcome feelings and the recollection of painful memories and may not be in a place where they are ready to process the unearthed memories or unwelcomed feelings. During treatment, clients have a right to proceed as they wish, including not addressing events or feelings until they are ready The client should be provided with a safe space where they can share their concerns openly.

Voluntary Participation in Counseling

In most cases, clients elect to engage in counseling services. In the informed consent document, it is important to state that counseling requires a level of commitment with time, financial resources, and effort.

Client Participation

The informed consent should clearly state the expectations that the clinician has for the client. An example expectation would be that the client will arrive on time for the scheduled appointments and ready to talk. Another reasonable expectation is that the client will not be under the influence of any mind-altering chemicals or substances. The clinician should let the client know that to receive the most benefit from counseling, the client should be honest and forthcoming about experiences and feelings. The client needs to be made aware that they are expected to be actively involved in the decision-making and overall counseling process.

Clinician Participation

This is the opportunity for the clinician to give their view of human nature and the counseling process/relationship. The clinician can also use this point to clarify their theoretical orientation(s) and inform the client how they prefer to facilitate counseling, as well as what the client can expect from the clinician (i.e., timeliness, keeping appointments, respect for the client and their experience, etc.).

Clinician Qualifications, Credentials, and Special Interests

The clinician should state their clinical qualifications to provide counseling services, followed by specialized training, certifications, and research interests. Just as in the section for clinician participation, this section can also discuss the clinician's approach to therapy and theoretical orientation.

Supervision and/or Consultation with Colleagues

Of course, if a clinician is not independently licensed, there will need to be a supervision disclosure. The supervisor's name, credentials, and contact information must be disclosed in the informed consent document. It is also wise to list the expected length of supervision and a brief description and frequency of supervisory meetings. This disclosure is meant to explain the supervisory relationship to the client. This is so the client can be aware of the supervisor and their role in supervising the clinician's work and the client's overall treatment. Additionally, it is common practice to consult with colleagues, especially when a clinician is unsure of how to assist a client or handle a specific situation that may occur during counseling. It is sound to let the client know that even though a consultation with a colleague may occur, the clinician will maintain the client's confidentiality by excluding the client's name or identifying information.

Length of Counseling

The clinician should provide a general plan regarding the frequency the client may be asked to schedule appointments, as well as the length of each meeting. For example, the informed consent may note, "We will meet every week or every other week at a mutually agreed-upon time for 45 minutes, but meetings may occasionally run as long as 50–60 minutes. The length of your session may vary based on need and we will reevaluate our initial plan monthly."

Privilege, Confidentiality, and Exceptions to Confidentiality

The information shared in counseling will remain confidential, and stating that clearly on the informed consent is imperative. Client–clinician privilege must be mentioned as well. This means that the clinician is not required to testify or speak in court or to other attorneys without specific permission from the client, a waiver of right to privilege, or a court order/subpoena. There are exceptions to confidentiality, which vary by state. Some examples of limits to confidentiality include (a) reasonable suspicion of the client's involvement in abuse or neglect of a child or vulnerable adult or that they are a victim of child abuse or elder abuse; (b) if the client is taking illicit drugs and is pregnant; (c) if the client is a danger to themselves or others (suicidal/homicidal); (d) if the client has reported sexual misconduct with a different clinician; and (e) if a judge orders the client's records.

Limitations to confidentiality must be discussed with the client in full disclosure. Additional limitations to confidentiality occur when the client is a minor and a parent or guardian has the legal right to access the underage client's records (please refer to your state laws for individualized specifics).

Providing Therapy to Minors

Every clinician must have a statement in their informed consent document that addresses the complexities of providing counseling to minor clients. In most cases and states, custodial parents must sign an agreement for services for the minor child. In the case of divorced parents, parents who no longer live together, or where legal custody is shared or split, each (shared) custodial parent must agree to services and must do so prior to the minor being seen by the clinician. Disclosure about how records and treatment plans for minors are stored and the rights of the legal parents to their minor children's records vary from state to state, so it is imperative to consult your state laws.

STATEMENT TO MINOR CLIENTS

Clinicians should always treat minor clients as individuals, with rights. In the informed consent form, clinicians need to document how they address the minor client's documentation and parent/guardian involvement, which can aid in building rapport between the therapist and the minor client. Another way to aid in helping the client develop trust is explaining how the clinician manages the triad of counselor, minor client, and parents/guardians. A simple statement such as "If you are under the age of 18 years, the law gives your parents the right to review your records" may be helpful for minor clients. This may also forge an opportunity that permits a discussion of what all the documentation entails.

Payment, Fees, and Insurance

It is critical that payment expectations be outlined in the informed consent. Hourly rates, a sliding scale, application of insurance benefits, no-show fees, and any other possible monetary implications must be disclosed. If a clinician does not accept insurance, this must also be noted. It should also be disclosed to the client that most insurance companies require clinical diagnosis for insurance benefits to apply. In the case of a client using insurance to pay for therapeutic services, it is important to note that the insurance company may require copies of treatment plans, case notes, and outcomes. In the instance of a client utilizing a third-party payer for counseling services, a clinician cannot guarantee confidentiality, and this should be noted in the informed consent as a limit of confidentiality.

Client Records

A case file is compiled for every client. Intake information, assessments, treatment plans, and so on are to be kept in the client's case file. Clients need to be made aware of the protocol for storing and handling their records. This information should be disclosed in the informed consent document. In this section of the informed consent document, it is a good idea to have a clear statement outlining what types of records are kept, how the transferring of records is handled, how and when releases of information are needed, and the client's right to obtain their own records. The client should also be made aware of the length of time that a clinician will store the records, post-counseling termination, and how records will be handled if the clinician passes away before the records are scheduled to be disposed of.

Ethical Guidelines

A clinician should always follow specific ethical codes and legal statutes. It is important that the clinician disclose which ethical standards they uphold in the informed consent. Directions for obtaining copies of ethical guidelines and associated information should be stated if the client desires to review the ethical codes.

Termination

The end of the counseling relationship is natural and inevitable. Termination of the counseling relationship can bring up a variety of feelings for the client. Clinicians should be preparing the client for termination from the first counseling engagement. It is wise to include a statement about how termination will occur in the informed consent document. This can provide an opportunity for a conversation regarding discharge early in the counseling process. How termination is addressed will be specific to the client, but it is important to include a general statement about termination.

Evaluation or Client Satisfaction Survey

Clinicians practice due diligence by providing the client with a post-treatment evaluation or satisfaction survey. This is an appropriate practice of customer service, and it gives the client the ability to provide feedback on the services they have received.

The informed consent process is a way of managing risk for clinicians and their respective agencies, but the most important outcome of the informed consent process is to convey to clients that they will receive the services outlined in the informed consent document in the most ethical and professional way. If clinicians embrace this mindset while creating their informed consent document, they will lay the essential foundation for a successful practice and positive client outcomes.

CONCLUSION

Informed consent is legally and ethically required in mental health counseling. Informed consent focuses on client autonomy but also incorporates the principles of autonomy, beneficence, nonmaleficence, justice, and fidelity. Informed consent is not just a document included in a client's file; it is also a process that changes based on a variety of factors. Special consideration must be given when creating the document when working with marginalized populations, minors, and adults who are incapacitated. In developing an informed consent form, the clinician must be attentive to craft a multidimensional and thorough document about themselves and their expertise, the services that may be offered, and the responsibilities of the client and counselor in therapeutic alliance.

REFERENCES

An Act to Define the Age of Consent for Alcohol or Drug Treatment and Mental Health Services. Sec. 1. 22 MRSA §1502 (1995). https://legislature.maine.gov/legis/bills/bills_128th/billtexts/HP082601.asp

American Counseling Association. (2014). *2014 ACA code of ethics.* https://www.counseling.org/docs/default-source/default-document-library/2014-code-of-ethics-finaladdressc97d33f16116603abcacff0000bee5e7.pdf?sfvrsn=5d6b532c_6

American Psychological Association. (2017). *Ethical principles of psychologists and code of conduct.* https://www.apa.org/ethics/code

American Psychological Association. (2021, December 10). *New billing disclosure requirements take effect in 2022.* https://www.apaservices.org/practice/legal/managed/billing-disclosure-requirements

Dalal, K. P. (2020). Consent in psychiatry: Consent, application and implication. *Indian Journal of Medical Research, 151*(1), 6–9. https://doi.org/10.4103/ijmr.IJMR_1518_19

Ekmekci, P. E., & Arda, B. (2017). Interculturalism and informed consent: Respecting cultural differences without breaching human rights. *Cultural, 14*(2), 159–172. https://www.ncbi.nlm.nih.gov/pmc/articles/PMC5890951/

National Association of School Psychologists. (2020). *The professional standards of the National Association of School Psychologists.* https://www.nasponline.org/x55315.xml.

National Association of Social Workers. (2021). *Code of ethics of the National Association of Social Workers.* https://www.socialworkers.org/About/Ethics/Code-of-Ethics/Code-of-Ethics

Quinn, S. C., Garza, M., Butler, J., & Fryer, C. S., Casper, E. T., Thomas, S., Barnard, D., & Kim, K. (2013). Improving informed consent with minority participants: Results from Research and Community Survey. *Journal of Empirical Research on Human Research Ethics, 7*(5), 45–55.

Tham, J., Gomez Garcia, A., & Garasic, D. M. (2022). *Cross-cultural and religious critiques of informed consent.* Routledge. https://library.oapen.org/bitstream/handle/20.500.12657/51388/9781000510386.pdf?sequence=1

World Population Review. (2024). *Age of consent for mental health treatment by state 2024.* Retrieved January 8, 2024, from https://worldpopulationreview.com/state-rankings/age-of-consent-for-mental-health-treatment-by-state

CHAPTER 4

Release of Information

Marisa White, PhD, Mona Gallo, EdD, Darlene Vaughn, PhD, and Gregory L. Bohner, PhD

INTRODUCTION

This chapter provides information on the practice of gaining permission from a client or guardian to communicate with, as well as what may be shared with, a variety of stakeholders in the lives of most clients served. The "how" and "when" to consider obtaining a release of information (ROI) is tremendously important because when providing mental health services, ROIs are required for any nonemergency communication with noncustodial parents and supporters, providers of other or previous services, judicial and legal institutions, medical providers, and so on. Most clients have the choice to disclose information or not; however, if a guardian is involved, it is their permission that is required.

The informed consent document may reference the ROI document as it pertains to confidentiality and privacy. Discussing this information can be beneficial to the clinical process because it communicates the clinician's commitment to confidentiality and the limits of confidentiality. It also informs the client about how their information will/may be used if they consent to an ROI. Understanding the precautions taken prior to releasing information assists in building therapeutic rapport by helping the client understand the importance of confidentiality and privacy.

When clinicians learn that their clients have a professional relationship with other mental health professionals, they will request an ROI from the client to inform the other professionals in an effort to establish positive and collaborative professional relationships to benefit the client (American Counseling Association [ACA], 2014). For example, if the client saw a clinician 3 years ago, that record may be informative for the client's current treatment. The clinician would request that the client sign a completed ROI and send it to the previous clinician. If part of the client's mental health services include medication and the client is receiving this adjunct treatment outside of the clinician's place of employment, then an ROI would be completed as a means for both service providers to communicate about the details of the client's needs.

If the client is receiving services from a treatment team, several providers within the same agency, then an ROI is not necessary, as long as the informed consent indicates the clinician's or agency's policy on a treatment team approach to client services. In addition, if the client previously received services within the same agency but with a different clinician, then an ROI from the client is not necessary. The rationale is the client is a client of the agency, not the clinician, and a new clinician would be expected to access the client's records as a part of the continuity of care provided by the agency.

In instances when clients have received prior mental health treatment and records cannot be obtained, it is imperative to consider the level of legal liability in deciding whether to work with a client or not (Baird, 2005). In cases where the client has a history of mental health treatment, whether directly prior to the current request for services or there is a distant history of mental health treatment, a clinician is advised to obtain an ROI from the client for their records from previous mental health treatment experiences. If the client is uncooperative or hesitant to allow for the ROI for records regarding previous mental health treatment, this may raise the level of concern for the clinician. Previous mental health treatment data can be a source of guidance in understanding the client's presenting concerns and providing current treatment. If the clinician requests an ROI for records and the client declines the request, then the clinician should document this request and the client's refusal and then evaluate the level of liability in working with a client who declines to allow previous mental health treatment to inform their current mental health treatment.

There are instances when a client's self-report can be an unreliable source of information—yes, even regarding their own data. There can be many reasons clients may not be able to remember their own information, including but not limited to mental status, substance use, injury, illness, trauma, age, or length of time since experiences occurred. In addition, when one is living their own life, memories can become commingled, which may make it difficult to distinctly discern dates, periods of time, seasons of life, situations, events, or people. In cases where the clinician believes the client's recollection of information is hampered, a request for an ROI may be beneficial and applicable to speak with the stakeholders in the client's life.

ETHICAL REASONS FOR A RELEASE OF INFORMATION

An ROI is a document that allows the client to dictate what information is shared with others. The ROI is used to obtain information from or to release information to an additional party. This form has both legal and ethical implications and involves informed consent and confidentiality, two cornerstones of mental health treatment. Documenting the client's consent to release information is an ethical necessity.

Clinicians need to take precautions to ensure the confidentiality of all information transmitted through the use of any medium, and when consulting about a client case with colleagues, they do not disclose confidential information that reasonably could lead to the identification of the client or other people or organizations with whom they have a confidential relationship unless they have obtained the prior consent of the person or organization or if the disclosure cannot be avoided. Any information that is disclosed is only to be to the extent necessary to achieve the purposes of the consultation (ACA, 2014; American Psychological Association, 2017).

Privacy and confidentiality are essential. Specifically, the ethical responsibility of a clinician is to protect client information, follow rules regarding when it can be released, and follow the proper steps when releasing it. A clinician may disclose confidential information when the client or authorized representative permits. Prior to disclosing client information, even by client consent, the clinician should inform the client of what will be disclosed and any potential consequences of such disclosure. If a clinician must disclose information, it is important to follow the minimum share rule and limit the amount of information shared to what is necessary to achieve the desired purpose (National Association of Social Workers, 2021).

As referred to in Chapter 3, client consent is an ongoing process. The ROI is a great example of how a clinician will continuously revisit consent with the client. The ROI document provides clients with the power to consent to what information can be shared, outside of emergency circumstances, with other individuals. Outside of obtaining an ROI at the beginning of treatment to attain information from a previous mental health provider, clinicians may also obtain an ROI at other points in treatment. For example, a clinician may want additional information when developing a treatment plan with a client because the desired information will provide information about learning or developmental disorders. In these cases, an ROI can specify that the previous information can be released to the current clinician.

A clinician may also use an ROI to provide information about a previous or current client to others. If a clinician wants to collaborate with other professionals about the care of a client, they will need the client's consent through an ROI. There are a variety of ways that this could be helpful to a mental health treatment provider. For example, a clinician may want to collaborate with a school counselor about the treatment of a client who is a minor. A clinician may want a family member to attend a session or to speak with a member of the client's support system. This would require the clinician to have the client's consent to communicate with these individuals.

LEGAL RATIONALE FOR THE ROI DOCUMENT

Like medical information, mental health data is protected by state and federal laws. The Health Insurance Portability and Accountability Act [HIPAA] of 1996 is one law that serves to safeguard individuals' protected health information (PHI) while also ensuring the smooth flow of health care information necessary for providing continuity of care. In short, it protects health care information from being shared with people who do not "need" the information to treat the client, including other providers. Mental health clinicians must comply with the strict regulations regarding the use and disclosure of PHI. This includes how information is handled in records, billing information, and any other data that could identify an individual's health status or the health care services received.

Under HIPAA (1996), the ROI is tightly controlled to protect clients' privacy rights. Generally, PHI can only be disclosed with the client's explicit authorization—through an ROI document. However, there are exceptions, such as for emergencies, treatment, payment, and health care operations. HIPAA requires clinicians to strike a delicate balance between protecting individuals' privacy and facilitating the efficient exchange of health care information necessary for quality care. When releasing information, HIPAA mandates certain protocols to ensure confidentiality. This includes measures such as securely transmitting data online, limiting access to only authorized personnel, and obtaining written consent when necessary (U.S. Department of Health and Human Services, 2022).

Since 1975 the rights of substance use treatment recipients have been protected by Part 2 of Title 42 of the Code of Federal Regulations (Part 2; Confidentiality of Substance Use Disorder Patient Records, 2024). This lesser known law focuses on the confidentiality of substance use disorder client records and outlines strict guidelines regarding information released that is related to the substance use disorder treatment. These regulations were designed to add an extra level of protection for individuals seeking treatment for substance abuse. Like HIPAA, Part 2 requires written consent prior to treatment, outlines limitations of privacy, and dictates confidentiality safeguards taken by the provider/clinician. Specifically, Part 2 identifies the need for consent and indicates that the consent to release information must specify what information can be shared, with whom, and for what purpose. It also indicates that clinicians must provide confidentiality safeguards (storage and transmission protocol) and explain the expectations of privacy (medical emergencies and when mandated by law) to clients (Confidentiality of Substance Use Disorder Patient Records, 2024).

Another law to consider is the Family Educational Rights and Privacy Act ([FERPA]. 1974). This law primarily applies to clinicians working in educational institutions, such as those providing services to students in elementary through college counseling and psychological services centers. Any records maintained by a clinician who is providing services in an educational institution are considered FERPA treatment records and are subject to disclosure rules according to FERPA guidelines as opposed to the HIPAA Privacy Rule (U.S. Department of Health and Human Services & U.S. Department of Education, 2019). Clinicians must obtain a written ROI from students to share the records with anyone who is not providing treatment. However, once this occurs, the records no longer qualify as treatment records and are viewed as educational records. For example, if a student asks a clinician in the counseling center to provide documentation to a disability resources office for academic accommodations, the information released to the disability resources office is then considered to be part of the student's educational record and is no longer protected as if it were a treatment record. The consent process becomes important in verifying students understand what is happening with their information.

Understanding the legal reasons behind completing and taking care of documentation not only helps clinicians be informed about their responsibilities but also helps them inform the clients of their rights in treatment. It should be noted that failure to comply with HIPAA and/or C.F.R. 42 (Part 2) regulations can result in severe penalties that include substantial fines, license revocation, and even criminal charges in cases of deliberate or negligent breaches of patient privacy.

DATA IN AN ROI

An ROI document typically contains personal information, purpose of the release, information to be released, duration of the release, procedures to revoke consent, the signature and date of the client, and a witness's signature. Personal information should include the name of the person releasing the information (clinician/agency) and the information regarding to whom it is released (receiving party), including the name, address, and contact details. The purpose will likely indicate if the clinician is obtaining information from another source, releasing information to another source, or exchanging information with another source. It is important to note the purpose of the ROI, which may include coordination of care, personal/client request, legal/court request, or emergency contact. Information released could range from the entire record to specific information about treatment (e.g., appointment dates, therapy notes, assessment data, diagnosis, discharge summary, etc.). The ROI document may specify that the client indicates the dates of the information that they want released (a specific period of time, such as 5/2023–current). The duration of the release could be a one-time authorization or ongoing consent. If there is ongoing consent provided, the ROI is often reviewed annually to ensure correctness. In addition, many states have laws in place designating the timeframe of a valid ROI before a new one would need to be obtained from the client. Ongoing consent may be desired if the clinician thinks that they may need to contact the other party on more than one occasion. At any time, the client has the legal right to revoke consent. The ROI should outline the process to proceed if the client wishes to withdraw their consent. And it is wise to provide the client with a copy of the signed ROI for their reference and records.

It is important to note that an ROI does not provide the clinician with complete discretion for sharing unlimited information. Laws and ethical codes indicate that clinicians should take precautions when sharing information. As with informed consent, the consent to release information should be more than an arbitrary form. It is important that the client understands the benefits and risks of consenting to the release of information. It is also important to indicate what information is shared, to whom, and for what purpose.

CONCLUSION

An ROI is required for any stakeholder information sharing in mental health service provision. As with all other forms, an ROI document may differ depending on the agency, state, clinician, client population, and so on. Some ROI forms have check boxes that a client can select to determine what information is or is not disclosed. Other forms are more general and only provide a line for the client to indicate what they decide or decline to share. Most ROI documents have headings that organize the necessary information into specific sections. This can help the reader understand the important information being requested or being shared. Completion of ROI may occur in the organizational and clinical intake or at any time thereafter as needed. Whoever is designated to establish the client in the organizational recordkeeping system provides the emergence of actual service delivery and the start of the clinical assessment.

REFERENCES

American Counseling Association. (2014). *2014 ACA code of ethics*. https://www.counseling.org/docs/

American Psychological Association. (2017). *Ethical principles of psychologists and code of conduct*. https://www.apa.org/ethics/code

Baird, B. (2005). *The internship, practicum and field placement handbook: A guide for the helping professions* (4th ed.). Routledge.

Confidentiality of Substance Use Disorder Patient Records, 42 C.F.R. § 2 (2024).

Family Educational Rights and Privacy Act of 1974, 20 U.S.C. § 1232g (1974).

Health Insurance Portability and Accountability Act, Pub. L. No. 104-191, § 264, Stat. 1936 (1996).

National Association of Social Workers. (2021). *Code of ethics of the National Association of Social Workers.* https://www.socialworkers.org/About/Ethics/Code-of-Ethics/Code-of-Ethics

U.S. Department of Health and Human Services. (2022, October 20). *Individuals' right under HIPAA to access their health information.* https://www.hhs.gov/hipaa/for-professionals/privacy/guidance/access/index.html

U.S. Department of Health and Human Services & U.S. Department of Education. (2019, December). *Joint guidance on the application of FERPA and HIPAA to student health records.* https://www.hhs.gov/sites/default/files/2019-hipaa-ferpa-joint-guidance.pdf

CHAPTER 5

Intake Assessment Documentation

*Darlene Vaughn, PhD, Mona Gallo, EdD, Holly J. Mattingly, PhD,
Gregory L. Bohner, PhD, and Daniel R. Romero, PhD*

INTRODUCTION

Clinical assessment is a segment of the intake process where the clinician interviews the client for the first time to gain information while concurrently developing a new and fragile relationship with the client (Gill et al., 2014; Whiston, 2017). The clinical assessment begins with awareness. Awareness may come as a formal referral from a community entity, a concerned individual, or the client who makes the request themselves (Ivey et al., 2018). Once the client presents for counseling services, information-gathering begins that will include an intake, a clinical assessment, and a mental status exam. In the initial interview clinicians gather basic client information and use assessment tools to explore the client's presenting issues (Gill et al., 2014; Whiston, 2017). After the clinician has completed the clinical interview, they utilize the client's background information to determine which additional assessment instruments or strategies are significant for the client (Sheparis et al., 2020).

ETHICAL REASONS FOR ASSESSMENT

The counseling, social work, and psychology professional ethical codes all consider and address the necessity and process of assessment. A primary purpose of educational, mental health, psychological, and career assessment is to gather information related to the client for a variety of purposes that include but are not limited to client decision-making, diagnosis, treatment planning, and forensic proceedings. The assessment process may include both qualitative and quantitative methodologies.

Clinicians should be able to provide an accurate description of the purpose, norms, validity, reliability, and applications of the procedures and any special qualifications of assessment instruments and their use (American Counseling Association [ACA], 2014). Assessment instruments should be valid and reliable for the population being assessed (ACA, 2014; American Psychological Association [APA]. 2017). However, if validity and reliability of an assessment instrument has not been demonstrated, then the clinician should provide a description of the advantages and constraints of the findings and interpretation provided (APA, 2017). Clinicians are to use evaluative practices that are current and used for professional reasons, report any results accurately (National Association of Social Workers [NASW], 2021), and to conduct, modify, score, interpret, or employ assessments that are appropriate and applicable, and with the correct application (APA, 2017). It is important to remember that clinicians should only provide testing and assessment services that they have received trained for and are competent in providing (ACA, 2014; APA, 2017; NASW, 2021).

Clinicians are advised to retrieve voluntary informed consent (ACA, 2014; APA, 2017; NASW, 2021) and to educate clients during the informed consent process that there is the possibility of being reassessed as part of the counseling process (ACA, 2014). Prior to beginning any assessment, it is imperative for the assessor to provide an explanation of the assessment instrument and the nature and purposes of assessment, as well as the specific use of results by potential recipients (ACA, 2014; APA, 2017). Once the client (or legally authorized person) consents to the parameters of the counseling relationship, the assessment process, and other pertinent counseling related engagement, the clinician can then proceed with the assessment process (Ivey et al., 2018; Sheparis et al., 2017).

During the assessment process, clinicians consistently maintain their ethical responsibility to those being assessed and consider the client's personal and cultural contexts (ACA, 2014; APA, 2017). The assessor should approach this process in the terms and language that the client (or other legally authorized person on behalf of the client) can understand (ACA, 2014; APA, 2017; NASW, 2021). Ethical clinicians use caution when selecting and using evaluation techniques that were developed using populations that differ from the client. Clinicians also recognize the historical and social prejudices in the misdiagnosis and pathologizing of certain individuals and groups and strive to raise awareness of and to address such biases in themselves or others. To mitigate these concerns, counselors must use thorough and appropriate assessment techniques to provide a proper diagnosis of mental disorders (ACA, 2014; APA, 2017).

Clinicians are to make sure that an assessment does not create unreasonable distress, peril, or hardship for the client (NASW, 2021). And lastly, clinicians allow the person being assessed to end the assessment at any time. If the client chooses to end an assessment, it is advised that the clinician inform the client of any potential consequences of ending the assessment (ACA, 2014; APA, 2017; NASW, 2021).

LEGAL REASONS FOR ASSESSMENT

The objective of an intake with each new client is to assess the client's concerns and determine the most appropriate treatment approach that best suits the client's needs (Griffin, 2022). Most mental health facilities or agencies use standardized forms to gather the client's initial information for the case file. The person who provides an intake for clinical services with a client is dependent on the policies and procedures of the mental health setting. The intake may occur in person or consist of mailing, emailing, or using a client portal where the expectation is for the client to independently complete many of their own intake documents. An organizational intake may be facilitated by a designated intake worker, a bachelor-level professional with specific training in the process of client intake, or be conducted by the clinician who will directly provide services to the client. Whoever manages the intake is responsible for ensuring the documentation was properly recorded in the client's case file.

Intake assessment requires the client's background information, their basic medical history, and current level of functioning (APA, 2017). Legally, clinicians must recognize the age, culture, disability, ethnic group, gender, race, language preference, religion, spirituality, sexual orientation, and socioeconomic status of clients and the cumulative effects on test administration and interpretation, placing test results in proper perspective with other relevant factors (ACA, 2014). The issues that clients share in any clinical interaction may be exacerbated by societal dysfunction, harassment, and oppression (Ivey et al., 2018). During the initial interview and assessment phase, pertinent information on difficulties the client has been experiencing can provide information that will influence treatment, clinical decision-making, the prioritization of issues being addressed, referrals, client prognosis, and intervention modalities (Whiston, 2017). Taken together, this affords the clinician the information needed to establish the need for treatment, the empirically based treatment modalities, and techniques to be utilized (ACA, 2014).

The selection of the assessment instruments should include a careful consideration of the validity, reliability, psychometric limitations, and appropriateness of instruments, and, when possible, it is best to use multiple forms of assessment, data, and/or instruments in forming conclusions, diagnoses, or recommendations (ACA, 2014). Documentation of the assessment needs to include the date and time of the assessment, the findings from the assessment, and the duration of time that the findings of the assessment would be considered valid. Assessments of clients need to be complete and accurate, document the clinician's decision-making process, outline how a diagnosis has been developed, include results of and receipt of testing, and include a description of following actions taken (Healthcare Providers Service Organization, 2019). A clinician's failure to do so by not knowing, neglect, or intent can result in legal ramifications.

With the composite of details in the assessment/evaluation details and clinical relationship, potential legalities abound. Laws, regulations, standards, policies, and rules exist to protect the client in any clinical relationship. It is the responsibility of the clinician to be familiar with the multiplicity of legal oversights for their profession and to ensure the services they provide follow established guidelines and protect the client. Responsible clinicians engage in methods of practice, such as thorough assessment and documentation, for clients and their own protection and, if needed, a legal defense.

INTAKE ASSESSMENT

A client intake assessment can include the use of many different documents. The clinician generally conducts a client intake with foundational documents that include a biopsychosocial interview and a mental status exam. Clinicians may choose to use brief versions of these forms, or more expanded versions. Clinicians may also choose to use different assessments instruments, however the choices of documents utilized during a client's intake may vary depending on the client's presenting state, the clinician's place of employment, and the clinician's experience.

Biopsychosocial Intake

The purpose of the clinical assessment is to provide accurate and dependable information about a person's emotional and mental health, all of which helps a clinician in decision-making, determining the diagnosis and differential diagnoses, and developing a plan of treatment (Weiner, 2004). Clinical assessment encompasses an application of assessment procedures that are to assess areas of need, diagnose a mental disorder, plan appropriate interventions, monitor counseling progress, and evaluate counseling outcomes (Sheparis et al., 2020). The clinical assessment can consist of an array of methods and instruments used to evaluate the client's functioning in multiple areas to inform and facilitate decisions or recommendations intended to improve functioning in one or more areas (Carlson, 2016). However, a standard format for clinical assessment is the biopsychosocial (BPS) interview and assessment approach (Nishioka et al., 2023).

The BPS originated within the 1970s medical community and has been adapted to facilitate a more thorough and holistic examination of clients. Generally, questions in the BPS include the client's perspective of their presenting problem or reason for the clinical visit, their health and medication histories, emotional issues, mental conditions (past and present), family of origin's health and social issues, and their work, education, social, and relational experiences (Nishioka et al., 2023). Some of the dimensions of the health and medical conditions may include relevant family history of past and current physical illness, a history and the status of the client's lifestyle choices, which may or may not include regular physical, dental, and eye checkups, tobacco and caffeine use, exercise, and diet. Sleep patterns and the client's last physical examination should be included in the data retrieved. The clinician should encourage the client to seek out an appointment with their primary care provider to rule out any physiological contributing factors related to the client's mental health concerns (Baird, 2005; Piazza & Baruth, 1990).

The process of gathering assessment information goes far beyond the formal use of assessment instruments and testing. Clinical assessment may assist the clinician with coordination of care with other care professionals, make decisions about client and public safety, determine referral and additional service needs, and identify course of treatment options (Gehart, 2016). Assessment information may be obtained from the client, stakeholder reports, and the clinician's observations. Assessment documentation is more thorough when the assessed domains not only include the client's history, beliefs, and dysfunction but also address the client's strengths and resources (Baird, 2005; Piazza & Baruth, 1990).

In a systematic approach, clinical assessment involves obtaining and documenting information about a person's conditions, symptoms, personal history, behavior, functioning, values, preferences, goals, and other relevant information (Oregon Health Care Association, 2017). Throughout the assessment interview, the clinician may need to respectfully inquire about cultural differences with the client, requesting clarity on gender, race, ethnicity, religion, or other cultural factors (Sheparis et al., 2020). The information that has been gathered is then analyzed through the clinician's clinical reasoning to identify the potential underlying causes of conditions and symptoms and then to choose appropriate interventions (Oregon Health Care Association, 2017). The outcome of a clinical assessment is intended to provide a thorough understanding of the client served; the impact of any identified disorder on the client's daily life, work, and social functioning; and the client's general well-being (Jull et al., 2008).

A *psychological assessment* would include the client's motivation for treatment, emotional status, level of functioning, cognitive capacity, and history of treatment received, including any difficulties or unsuccessful completions. *Social and family assessment* may include the client's current and previous family history (e.g., parents, siblings, living situation outside of family of origin, family dynamics, family history of illnesses, suicide, etc.), developmental history, and social status and functioning. The *social assessment* would address avocational activities and interests, peers, and recreational and leisure activities, while the *vocational and educational assessment* covers information about the client's employment and academic history to include their strengths and achievements. A *drug and alcohol assessment* would include data related to the client's history of use and misuse of prescribed, licit, and illicit substances, or lack thereof. In addition to asking the individual about substance use and misuse, age of first use, their 24-hour record, and signs of dependence, any family history of substance use can inform the clinician of a history of trauma (Baird, 2005; Piazza & Baruth, 1990).

It is imperative for the clinician to have knowledge of basic developmental issues and be able to structure an appropriate clinical interview because a positive correlation exists between the attention provided to the client's presenting concerns and effective outcomes (Whiston, 2017). Although the client's presenting problem information may be provided by a referral source, the clinician's inquiry to the client's identified need in relation to the visit starts the BPS and dimensional assessment process. Through a process of asking open-ended questions, expansive sharing may occur, but clinicians need to focus on relevant information (Ivey et al., 2018; Whiston, 2017). There is a need to recognize the totality and multiplicity of client issues. Defining the problem too narrowly may become a liability, so the clinician is encouraged to be open-minded to alternate descriptions that increase the potential for maneuverability, adaptability, and creativity in providing treatment (Gehart, 2016).

Biopsychosocial-Spiritual Intake

An addition to the BPS format is the inclusion of spirituality. Proponents of adding the spirituality dimension to the intake assessment have recognized that clinicians need to perform an accurate and adequate assessment of how clients relate to spirituality and religion and its impact or role in their lives. By including the exploration of spirituality and religion in the client's assessment, clinicians may glean insight into the impact spirituality and religion have had in the client's life, increasing the levels of sensitivity by the clinician to what gains clients may experience by revealing a deeply personal part of their inner world (Gill et al., 2014). Additionally, the inclusion of spirituality in the client's assessment may support subsequent clinical interpretations and decision-making (Gill et al., 2014; Oregon Health Care Association, 2017).

Like a general BPS, the *biopsychosocial-spiritual (BPSS) assessment* should include an assessment of the client's overall health. The clinician must be aware of the client's general health information and medical conditions to ensure there is no physiological basis for the client's presenting concerns (Whiston, 2017). Taking the time to ask the client about current and historical medical problems and problems with physical health may offer insight into their development and medical involvement (Gehart, 2016; Whiston, 2017). This part of the clinical interview includes inquiry into the client's birth and developmental history, illnesses and surgeries, medication(s) and side effects, sleep patterns, appetite, exercise regimen (or lack thereof), mood, pain, suicidal ideation, specific substance use, relationships and stability, intimate partner violence or abuse as victim or perpetrator, and significant life changes, such as loss, acquisitions, accomplishments, and improvements (Gehart, 2016; Whiston, 2017). Often, client statements may represent physical and emotional symptomatology, so it is imperative for the clinician to have a basic understanding of common medical issues and medications, including psychotropic medications, their use, and the correct spelling of the medication.

Clinicians need to inquire about the client's emotional and mental health. This exploration may include clinical queries regarding any previous diagnosis, first occurrence of symptoms, symptom severity, treatment, medication and side effect histories, any effects on sleep, appetite, weight, episodes of mood destabilization, any related hospitalizations, suicidal ideation and any attempts, any related substance use, violence, supportive relationships, and periods of emotional stability. It is imperative that clinicians ask clients about suicidality in clinical interactions and document the client's response. The same is true for asking about the client's risk for violence, especially if the client has demonstrated a lack of self-regulation, aggression, or victimization (Gehart, 2016; Whiston, 2017). Upon the completion of gathering the client's physical and mental health information, the clinician may seek to explore the client's symptomology potential and overall functioning by conducting a mental status exam.

Mental Status Exam

An informationally rich component of mental health inquiry is the *mental status exam (MSE)*, which may be facilitated by the long or mini-mental status exam (MMSE) formularies. Developed by Meyer in 1918, as cited by Voss and M Das (2022), the MSE became important to psychiatric diagnosing in standardizing a method to evaluate a patient's overall mental status (Johnson, 2018). By combining information gathered from passive observation during the interview with data acquired through direct questioning, an in-the-moment picture of the patient's mental status emerges (Voss & M Das, 2022). A full MSE is usually completed in initial sessions and then periodically or as needed by client presentation. Conversely, clinicians often use an MMSE as a matter of practice for checking in with the client at key times or in all sessions.

The MSE assessment supports the clinician in identifying signs and symptoms of mental illness and in making a diagnosis, as well as recognizing signs and monitoring symptoms throughout the treatment episode. The separate parts of the mental status

MSE look at different areas of mental functioning to thoroughly capture both the objective and subjective aspects of mental illness (Voss & M Das, 2022).

In the initial assessment, the MSE provides opportunities for the clinician to document the client's appearance and the client responses in demonstrating their current functioning. Areas covered include general awareness, orientation, attitude, speech, memory, intelligence, mood, behavior, cognitive processes, insight, judgment, and responsiveness (Whiston, 2017). The information may be documented on a checklist with clinician annotation or a short fill-in-the-blank form. Either format may capture a detailed snapshot of client's current presentation, which can inform the clinician of the client's current needs. The use of the MSE can expose information that may not have been offered by the client and/or guardian otherwise.

Conducting the MSE begins with a clinician's observations of the client. The clinician should document the client's apparent age and appearance, level of hygiene, and clothing selection and appropriateness for weather. The client's speech and pattern (normal, pressured, tangential, or circumstantial) is also observed and documented. The clinician will also observe and document the client's attitude and behavior (client presentation, whether the person is calm, cooperative, uncooperative, or belligerent). Additionally, clinicians observe and document the client's affect (normal range, broad, depressed, restricted, flat, labile, blunted, reactive, mood congruent, or tearful). Affect can include facial expression, body posture, and the congruence of client responses. The MSE will also include a place for the clinician to observe and document the client's thought process (whether the client is goal-directed and logical or disorganized, grandiose, perseverant, phobic, as well as the current or past presence of delusions and obsessions/compulsions). In addition, the clinician should query as to whether the client has experienced any visual, auditory, tactile, gustatory, olfactory, or spatial hallucinations. It is imperative to check to see if the client is suicidal and/or homicidal, has a history of suicidal ideation or plan, and if so, when and by what means, and document any attempts (Johnson, 2018; Sheparis et al., 2020; Whiston, 2017).

After the observational pieces of the MSE, the clinician may ask the client to perform tasks that are designed to appraise the client's current abilities and processes. These sections are designed to check the client's parameter of orientation. The clinician would ask the client to respond to questions, such as naming the current month, day, year, day of week, location, and purpose of clinical meeting. The MSE may also have a section related to the client's memory. Often, recent, remote memory or past events are examined through a series of questions or short activities. Usually following the examination of the client's short-term memory is a query regarding global questions related to examples of current events, the current president and governor, and simple geography questions, such as naming bordering states (Johnson, 2018; Sheparis et al., 2020; Whiston, 2017). A client's ability to concentrate can be examined as well. The clinician may ask the client to recite serial number sequencing, usually with 7s or 3s, spelling the word "world" forward and backward, and following a simple three-step command. Examination of the client's abstract thought may occur through requests for proverb interpretation. Lastly, the MSE may include an examination of the client's level of insight into their condition, as well as their judgment (Johnson, 2018; Sheparis et al., 2020; Whiston, 2017).

Details collected using an MSE may allow the clinician to gain additional insights from aspects such as the influence of family and environmental factors on the client. Even though services are often being sought after by an individual, the client's family experiences may strongly influence their life response and identified concerns in the past and/or present. To understand the role of the family in the client's life, the clinician should explore the family structure, patterns of interaction, family rules, roles, power dynamics, and cultural nuances. Collecting process data on family dynamics, strengths, patterns of conflict, boundaries, and alliances allows the clinician and client to inform the treatment planning process (Capuzzi & Stauffer, 2020). Gathering information on the client's marital status, whether they have any children (and number of pregnancies), and their families' health and mental history offers insights and may expose patterns about behaviors and conditions related to alcohol/drug use, anxiety, depression, violence, disordered eating, obesity, psychiatric problems, suicide, and other pertinent issues (Whiston, 2017). Acquiring the aforementioned data may provide psychological liberation from historical trauma and may be realized when the underlying causes and effects have been explored (Ivey et al., 2018).

Clients are often impacted by family and social influences that are unconsciously related to others through their perspectives, worldviews, and self-conceptualizations (Ivey et al., 2018). The client's experiences and performance in education and employment settings are also integral to the clinical assessment formulation. Inquiring about patterns, accomplishments, and problems in the client's educational and vocational experience offers a natural progression to the clinical interview and allows the client to share about their performance history and individual patterns of relational behaviors (Whiston, 2017). Peer groups and intimate relationships are strong influences on most clients and may aid or hinder the treatment process (Capuzzi & Stauffer, 2020). Including environmental factors as part of understanding the client, the clinician can transition the clinical interview questions to the client's belief systems and motivations for seeking clinical involvement.

Since the theme of an initial clinical assessment is that of holistic information-gathering, it is helpful to explore the client's intrinsic belief system about spirituality and/or religion. Realizing how indicators for spiritual or religious belief manifest in an individual's choices is helpful for client and clinician connection and the therapeutic alliance.

Clothing choices, makeup, hairstyles, jewelry, grooming, and an imaginatively endless assortment of other pathways or combinations may imply an individual's personal or spiritual beliefs and values (Gill et al., 2014). With clinical observations of the client's appearance, behaviors, verbal responses, and so on made throughout the interview, assumptions may be made, but it is still important for the clinician to ask the client to describe their beliefs on spirituality and religion, or a lack thereof.

Even with the life details already shared, the client may feel a level of discomfort, which is a normal experience. Some clients may respond negatively, self-blame, and deny any capabilities or lack recognition of strengths, but part of the intake assessment also addresses how the client interprets and reports on their perceived strengths. The clinician may decrease the client's discomfort by explaining that the question is multifaceted and includes their character, accomplishments, moments of resilience, survival, and success.

The same type of inquiry may be effective as the clinician asks about the areas of the client's life that they believe there is need for improvement. Since the clinical milieu is a collaboration between the clinician and client toward the client improving their life, the clinician should cooperate with what the client identifies as the areas they want to focus on for future sessions. Another natural progression may occur in the clinical interview as the clinician seeks to specifically identify the client's goal(s) for the counseling engagement. The clinician needs to directly ask the client what they want to accomplish while in treatment and then document the client's responses.

After completing the clinical interview, the clinician would utilize the client's background information to determine which additional assessment instruments or strategies are significant for the client (Sheparis et al., 2020). A clinician should select and cautiously use assessment techniques, recognizing the effects age, culture, disability, ethnic group, gender, race, language preference, religion, spirituality, sexual orientation, and socioeconomic status may have on test administration and interpretation. Clinicians place test results in proper perspective with other relevant factors. Furthermore, clinicians are careful in selecting testing instruments and consider the validity, reliability, psychometric limitations, and appropriateness of any instruments they are considering. When possible, clinicians are advised to use multiple forms of assessment and/or instruments in forming conclusions, diagnoses, or recommendations (ACA, 2014; APA, 2017; NASW, 2021). Appropriate testing examples include administering the Patient Health Questionnaire-9 to any client for general assessment, asking a person reporting experimental substance use to complete an age-appropriate Substance Abuse Subtle Screening Inventory, and administering the Edinburgh Postnatal Depression Scale to a new mother who reports recent patterns of crying, outbursts, and feelings of numbness.

After the completion of the clinical interview and any initial assessment instruments completed, there are several final steps for the clinician to take. Clinicians will, almost always, complete a diagnostic impression with a formally written diagnosis, which may include a provisional diagnosis, a formal diagnosis, and several differential diagnoses. Clinicians will also document a summarization of the clinical interview information and make treatment recommendations for client care.

THOROUGH DOCUMENTATION GUIDES TREATMENT CONSIDERATIONS

Thorough and thoughtful clinical documentation can lead to more accurate client treatment. Clients are best served in treatment when clinicians carefully consider developing an accurate diagnosis and view the client's presenting concerns from their cultural, social, and historical influences.

Diagnosis

Utilizing a plethora of clinical interview techniques, the clinician can then examine the criteria in the most recent edition of the American Psychiatric Association's ([APA], 2022) *Diagnostic and Statistical Manual of Mental Disorders* (5th ed., text rev. [*DSM–5-TR*]) to identify the client's potential mental disorder(s) and then progress toward a diagnosis(es). Using the *DSM-5-TR*, the clinician engages a dimensional approach to diagnosing the client's condition and the severity rating of any identified disorder while considering and including human development, multicultural issues, and behavior (Ivey et al., 2018; Sheparis et al., 2020).

Each mental disorder in the *DSM-5-TR* (APA, 2022) includes a list of diagnostic criteria (i.e., symptoms, emotions, behaviors, and cognitions) that must be met by the client for a diagnosis to be made. The diagnosis may then be specified with applicable features such as catatonia, seasonal patterns, anxious distress, or mood congruent psychosis. In the *DSM-5-TR* (APA, 2022), each disorder has descriptions of age of onset, cultural and gender-related components, prevalence, risk, lifetime patterns, predisposing factors, complications, familial patterns, and differential diagnosis (Sheparis et al., 2020).

Cultural and Historical Influences

It benefits the client when the clinician recognizes the cultural effects in the manner that the client's problems are defined and experienced while considering the client's socioeconomic and cultural experiences when diagnosing mental disorders. Exploring cultural differences is especially important to obtain clarification of the client's cultural norms. Recognizing and understanding the client's cultural differences can often inform the clinician of the client's behaviors and verbalizations. This may also aid clinicians in accepting beliefs in response to crises and aid in refraining from a premature and potentially incorrect diagnosis (Sheparis et al., 2020). It is the responsibility of each clinician to conservatively diagnose while remaining culturally competent and considering the cultural implications in the instrumentation employed and cultural frames of reference in the client's behaviors that were evaluated.

Special care is necessary in recognizing historical and social prejudices which have led to the misdiagnosis and pathologizing of certain individuals and groups. Clinicians need to strive to increase awareness of and to address such biases in themselves or others. Counselors need to provide proper diagnosis of mental disorders using assessment techniques (including personal interviews) to determine client care (e.g., locus of treatment, type of treatment, recommended follow-up) that are selected carefully and appropriately used. Lastly, clinicians may refrain from making and/or reporting a diagnosis if they believe that it would cause harm to the client or others. Clinicians need to carefully consider both the positive and negative implications of a diagnosis (ACA, 2014).

Clinicians need to complete rigorous training and incorporate a continuum of professional development opportunities to strengthen skills of observation, description, definition, documentation, and reporting information. Clinicians should strive to improve their knowledge base for assessing specific conditions and situations and providing correct interventions (Oregon Health Care Association, 2017).

Documentation

When the information gathered in the clinical assessment interview is documented into the client's record, the clinician retains immediate access to the wealth of details received from the client and eases the angst of creating the clinical assessment summary. The *clinical assessment summary* provides an overview of salient points of therapeutic consideration (i.e., opens with client's name, age, observed impressions, marital and legal status open the summary statement, followed by the client's unique needs, diversity factors, potential effects of treatment on the client, and any areas of client and clinician disagreement). The clinician will also include the client's identified stressors, protective factors, any testing completed with the matching results, the diagnostic impression, the client's current stage of change and a prognosis, the expected client outcome, and an assessment summary statement (Gehart, 2016). To complete the clinical assessment report, the clinician documents any recommendations and referrals identified through the assessment process.

It is best for the clinician to take an inclusive approach when making recommendations and referrals. For example, if the client has not had a recent physical examination by a physician, then the clinician should provide the client with a list of medical providers and/or a referral for an appointment may be made with the client's agreement. Clinicians also need to consider referrals related to the client's dental care needs and medication considerations. Other recommendations and referrals may occur regarding housing, utility assistance, transportation, and information on other necessary elements of optimal functioning. Once the clinician has shared the recommendations verbally with the client and documented them, the initial clinical assessment is complete.

CONCLUSION

The clinical assessment process is an essential part of building rapport with the client and any stakeholders involved in their care. The assessment process is generally part of the initial contact with the client and is essential in gaining foundational information related to the client's background, presenting and precipitating problems, as well as crucial data that may emerge using specific assessment instruments. The clinical assessment and intake process become key components in erecting a case conceptualization, treatment plan, as well as guiding the overall identification of the client's symptoms, diagnosis, problems, goals, and interventions.

EXAMPLE FORMS

The forms commonly used for clinical assessment are the BPS and the MSE. Please reference the two examples below. Also, remember that there are many different versions of these forms, and these are only two examples.

Biopsychosocial-Spiritual

BIOPSYCHOSOCIAL-SPIRITUAL INTAKE ASSESSMENT

Case Number __________ Client Name __________________________ Date ____________

Referred By ____

Emergency Contact Name/Phone ____

Identifying Data:

Age ______ Ethnic Background ________ Education ______________

☐ Single ☐ Widowed ☐ Married ☐ Divorced ☐ Separated ☐ Cohabiting

☐ Male ☐ Female

Employment Status __________________________ Employed As __________________________

PRESENTING ISSUES In client's own words, state the client's reason for seeking treatment/assistance at this time. ____

____

____

HISTORY OF PRESENT ISSUES Chronological narrative describing symptoms, impairment, and other data indicative of maladaptive/compulsive behaviors. Discuss precipitating events, intensity of symptoms, and duration of symptoms. This section should substantiate diagnoses: ______________________________

____

____

____

____

PHYSICAL AND MENTAL HEALTH HISTORY

Mental Health/Substance Abuse Treatment History (diagnosis, outpatient treatment, hospitalizations, treatment outcomes, etc.)

Client denies relevant history? ☐ Yes ☐ If present, elaborate ☐ No

____

____

____

Family history of mental health/substance use problems (e.g., phobias, suicide, suicide attempts, psychiatric hospitalizations, manic depressive illness, schizophrenia, violence, etc.; emphasize generational patterns).

Relevant family history? ☐ Yes ☐ No ☐ Unknown

____

____

____

Medical History

Currently under care of physician? ☐ Yes ☐ No Date of last physical exam ____________

Current medical problems ______________________________

____

Past medical problems ______________________________

____

Medications (prescription/nonprescription) ______________________________

____

DISABILITIES (nature of disability, if applicable, and identification of related needs and recommendations)

____

☐ Not applicable ☐ Daily living skills ☐ Supervision

☐ Independent living skills ☐ Leisure activities ☐ Health/safety

☐ Nutrition/dietary needs ☐ Need for assistive technology or prosthetic

Recommendations/Referrals ______________________________

____

PSYCHOSOCIAL INFORMATION

Marital/Significant Other ______________________________

____

Children (Note children 3 years or younger with developmental disabilities/delays) ____________

____

Parents ______________________________

____

Siblings ______________________________

____

Family Relationships (Describe childhood, home environment and family dynamics, including relationships with parents and how parents related to each other, violence in family, if any)

____

____

____

Social Information (Address social/leisure time and stress management activities)

____

____

____

Resources (Note family and social network as resources to client)

____

____

Education (Address status as well as success or failure) ______________________________

____

____

Legal (current status, any history as related to service needs) ______________________________

____

____

Cultural (Address any special treatment considerations related to cultural/racial background) __________

____

SPIRITUAL/RELIGIOUS ASSESSMENT (Describe client's current attendance, religious affiliation, and response to above, indicate client's satisfaction level with their spiritual involvement.)

____

____

NON-SUBSTANCE RELATED ADDICTIVE OR COMPULSIVE BEHAVIOR ASSESSMENT (Identify gambling, eating, sex, cleaning, shopping, internet, work, etc.)

Comments: ____

(Check appropriate problem areas)

☐ Not applicable ☐ Legal/financial problems

☐ Frequency ☐ Loss of control

SUICIDE/HOMICIDE ASSESSMENT

Client has:	PAST		PRESENT	
• Suicidal/homicidal thoughts	☐ Yes	☐ No	☐ Yes	☐ No
• Suicidal/homicidal urges	☐ Yes	☐ No	☐ Yes	☐ No
• Suicidal/homicidal plans	☐ Yes	☐ No	☐ Yes	☐ No
• Prior suicide attempts	☐ Yes	☐ No	☐ Yes	☐ No

Additional Comments ____

PHYSICAL/SEXUAL ABUSE ASSESSMENT

• Physical/sexual abuse	☐ Yes	☐ No	☐ Yes	☐ No
• Physical/sexually abusive	☐ Yes	☐ No	☐ Yes	☐ No

Yes to any of the above, describe and assess the following:

- Seriousness of intent
- Identified risks to client or potential victim
- Suicide attempts (methods, number of attempts, approximate dates)
- Actions taken/referrals made (e.g., hospitalization, second opinion, psychiatric evaluation, increase psychotherapy sessions per week, other)

____

____

____

____

STOP HERE. THE FOLLOWING PAGES ARE TO BE COMPLETED WITHOUT CLIENT INPUT. THEY ARE BASED SOLELY ON THE COUNSELOR'S OBSERVATION AND SHOULD BE FINISHED ASAP AFTER CONCLUSION OF INTAKE SESSION. THE FINAL PAGE INCLUDES A SIGNATURE BLOCK FOR THE CLIENT, COUNSELOR, AND SUPERVISOR.

MENTAL STATUS

General Appearance: A brief, concise, verbal portrait—physical characteristics, apparent age, dress, cleanliness, facial expression, eye contact, etc.: ______________________________

____

Affective State	☐ Appropriate to content	☐ Anxious	☐ Blunted
	☐ Flat	☐ Depressed	☐ Inappropriate
	☐ Labile	☐ Frightened	☐ Angry
	☐ Controlled	☐ Euphoric	☐ Irritable
	☐ Intense	☐ Calm	

☐ Other ______________________________

Attitude	☐ Pleasant	☐ Paranoid	☐ Introspective/Insightful/Intuitive
	☐ Hostile	☐ Motivated	☐ Seeks Direction
	☐ Sarcastic	☐ Not Motivated	☐ Uncooperative
	☐ Cooperative	☐ Distrusting	

☐ Other ______________________________

Motor Activity	☐ Unremarkable	☐ Agitated	☐ Gestures
	☐ Hypoactive	☐ Psychomotor	☐ Unusual Movements
	☐ Hyperactive	☐ Tics	☐ Abnormal Involuntary Movements

☐ Other ______________________________

Thought Process			
	☐ Intrusive Thoughts	☐ Rapid	☐ Pressured
	☐ Unremarkable	☐ Loose Associations	
	☐ Spontaneous	☐ Overly Detailed	☐ Flight of Ideas
	☐ Obsessive	☐ Circumstantial	☐ Blocking

☐ Other ______________________________

Thought Content

☐ Unremarkable ☐ Delusions ☐ Distortion

☐ Preoccupational ☐ Idea of Reference ☐ Hypochondriacal

☐ Hallucinations ☐ Guilt

☐ Other ______________________________

Orientation (time, place, person) Client is oriented Xs 3 ☐ Yes ☐ No

Memory Intact ☐ Yes ☐ No

Intelligence ☐ Below Average ☐ Average ☐ Above Average

Judgment ☐ Intact ☐ Impaired

Abstract Reasoning ☐ Adequate ☐ Inadequate

Additional Comments ______________________________

DIAGNOSTIC IMPRESSION

Primary ______________________________

Secondary ______________________________

Tertiary ______________________________

SUMMARY OF CLINICAL FORMULATION OF ISSUES AND TREATMENT RECOMMENDATIONS

____

____

____

____

____

____

Client Signature ______________________ **Date** ______________

Counselor Signature ______________________ **Date** ______________

Supervisor Signature and Credentials ______________ **Date** ______________

Mental Status Exam

MENTAL STATUS EXAM GUIDELINES	
CATEGORY	**EXAMPLES OF OBSERVATION DETAIL**
Appearance	• Is the person well-groomed or unkempt? • What is the person wearing? • Are clothes appropriate for weather and situation?
Speech	Is the person's speech normal, pressured, tangential, or circumstantial?
Attitude and Behavior	• Is the person calm, cooperative, uncooperative, or belligerent?
Mood	• Is the person's mood euthymic, irritable, elevated, anxious, or depressed?
Affect	• Is the person's affect within normal range, depressed, constricted, flat, labile, blunted, reactive and mood congruent, or tearful?
Thought Process and Content	• Is the person goal-directed and logical or disorganized? • Are there any delusions, phobias, or obsessions/compulsions? • Is the person suicidal and/or homicidal?
Orientation	• Is the person oriented to time and place?
Perception	• Did the person display signs of hallucinations or delusions during interview?
Memory	• Remote—can person remember past events? • Recent—can person remember 3/3 objects after 5 min? • Immediate—how well can the person perform digit span?
Fund of Knowledge	• Is the person aware of current events? Give examples. • Does the person know the names of the president and governor? • Can the person answer simple geography questions, such as naming bordering states?
Concentration	• Serial 7's or 3's. • Spell "world" forward and backward. • Is the person able to follow a three-step command?
Abstract Thought	• Is the person able to interpret proverbs?
Insight and Judgment	• Does the person have insight into their condition? • Does the person show good judgment (e.g., when asked what they would do if they smelled smoke in crowded theater)?

* The MSE must include detailed observations regarding the person's appearance, speech, attitude, behavior, mood, and affect. If not within normal limits, the MSE must also include detailed observations regarding the person's thought process and content, orientation, perception, memory, fund of knowledge, concentration, abstract thought, insight, and judgment.

THE CASE OF ABEL (ENTIRE CASE IN CHAPTER 2)

Abel, a 32-year-old male, comes to the intake session of counseling because he is "unhappy with how things are going in his marriage" and he cannot "figure out how to make things work." When Abel came to see you for the first session, he smiled and shook your hand and asked "How does this work?" He was restless and had a difficult time keeping his focus on the questions at hand. He reports that his wife, Mary, a 37-year-old White woman, does not listen to him and does not respect him. She constantly berates him, particularly in front of their 10-year-old son, Simon, and listens to her friends and family more than she listens to him. He is currently working as a truck driver in a local factory and is attending night classes to finish his associate's degree in accounting. His wife works as a hospital administrator. She is the primary breadwinner and provides them with a comfortable life, though they often argue about money. He also grew up in the Ethiopian Orthodox Tewahedo Church and wants Simon to attend church with him, while Mary grew up in a Reform Judaism synagogue and wants Simon to choose for himself.

Abel has told you that he is close to his mother, who has always been supportive of him, but has a tense relationship with his father. He was born in Ethiopia, but his family immigrated to Los Angeles when he was a teenager. He says that his father would berate him and call him "worthless." He says this is why he does not feel good about his work and does not think he can do anything to make people happy. He stopped caring about school until he got in trouble for egging his teacher's house in 10th grade. His family still lives in California, but his mother-in-law lives about 30 minutes away. She has never turned him away, but he thinks she was never happy that he married into the family, possibly because of his ethnicity. His father-in-law passed away 4 years ago.

Abel said that he will do well for a while, but every 9–12 months, he goes into a "funk." He does not like his work and just wants to sit in front of the TV all day long. He says this is when he gets into verbal fights with his wife, and these will sometimes turn physical (e.g., throwing pillows, punching walls, breaking decorations) which Abel says his wife can "dish it out" as well as he can. According to Abel, he is a passionate person, and his wife is cold and emotionless until they fight. These funks last for about a month and then he starts to feel better again. They originally started about 10 years ago, but he feels like they have gotten worse over the past few years because he has started having thoughts of killing himself. He said these are usually in the form of thinking that everyone would be better off if he was not around. As you discussed these thoughts further, he denied any hallucinations and did not exhibit any delusional thinking.

When asked about his physical health, Abel says he has never had any major surgeries and regularly does his annual physical. He exercises three to four times a week, though this decreases during a funk. Abel stated that he is classified as overweight but says that is because he eats out for lunch every day. He came from work and his clothes were neat and clean.

According to Abel, when he told his wife 6 months ago that he had been having suicidal thoughts for the past couple of years, she told him to do whatever he likes. He started to seriously contemplate killing himself, so he checked himself into a treatment hospital. When asked about how he would do so, he shrugs and says, "Probably drive somewhere so my son doesn't see me." He stayed at the hospital for 2 weeks and participated in group sessions and individual discussions about his life goals. As you continue to talk with Abel, he acknowledges who he is and can identify the current year and where you are meeting.

Abel is seeing you as follow-up treatment and to continue working on making his marriage and life "more bearable." He wants to figure out how to better communicate with his wife and take control of his thoughts for his little boy. He says that he has been feeling good lately, with no thoughts of suicide, and definitely doesn't want to hurt anyone else but wouldn't be surprised if a funk started soon. "I just really want to get on top of this, so it doesn't become a bigger issue."

MINI MENTAL STATUS EXAM

Client Name: Abel			**Date:** May 3, 2024		
OBSERVATIONS					
Appearance	☒ Neat	☐ Disheveled	☐ Inappropriate	☐ Bizarre	☐ Other
Speech	☒ Normal	☐ Tangential	☐ Pressured	☐ Impoverished	☐ Other
Eye Contact	☒ Normal	☐ Intense	☐ Avoidant	☐ Other	
Motor Activity	☐ Normal	☒ Restless	☐ Tics	☐ Slowed	☐ Other
Affect	☒ Full	☐ Constricted	☐ Flat	☐ Labile	☐ Other
Comments:					
MOOD					
☐ Euthymic	☒ Anxious	☐ Angry	☐ Depressed	☐ Euphoric	☐ Irritable ☐ Other
Comments:					
COGNITION					
Orientation Impairment	☒ None	☐ Place	☐ Object	☐ Person	☐ Time
Memory Impairment	☒ None	☐ Short-Term	☐ Long-Term	☐ Other	
Attention	☐ Normal	☒ Distracted	☐ Other		
Comments:					
PERCEPTION					
Hallucinations	☒ None	☐ Auditory	☐ Visual	☐ Other	
Other	☒ None	☐ Derealization	☐ Depersonalization		
Comments:					
THOUGHTS					
Suicidality	☒ None	☐ Ideation	☐ Plan	☐ Intent	☐ Self-Harm
Homicidality	☒ None	☐ Aggressive	☐ Intent	☐ Plan	
Delusions	☒ None	☐ Grandiose	☐ Paranoid	☐ Religious	☐ Other
Comments:					

BEHAVIOR					
☒ Cooperative	☐ Guarded		☐ Hyperactive	☐ Agitated	☐ Paranoid
☐ Stereotyped	☐ Aggressive		☐ Bizarre	☐ Withdrawn	☐ Other
Comments:					
INSIGHT	☒ Good	☐ Fair	☐ Poor	Comments:	
JUDGMENT	☐ Good	☐ Fair	☒ Poor	Comments:	

ADDITIONAL COMMENTS ______________________________

____

____

Counselor: Tara Pist, MEd **Date:** May 3, 2024

MENTAL STATUS EXAM

Client's Name: Abel Tesfaye **DOB:** 04/16/1992

APPEARANCE

Grooming: ☒ Normal ☐ Disheveled ☐ Unusual

Hygiene: ☒ Normal ☐ Body Odor ☐ Bad Breath ☐ Other______

MOTOR ACTIVITY

☐ Relaxed ☒ Restless ☐ Pacing ☐ Sedate

☐ Threatening ☐ Catatonic ☐ Posturing ☐ Mannerisms

☐ Tremors ☐ Tics ☐ Psychomotor Retardation

☐ Other______

INTERPERSONAL

☒ Cooperative ☐ Oppositional/Resistant

☐ Defensive ☐ Other______

SPEECH

☐ Characteristics ☒ Normal ☐ Slow ☐ Dysarthric

☐ Apraxic ☐ Pressured

☐ Expressive Language ☒ Normal ☐ Circumstantial ☐ Anomia

☐ Paraphasia ☐ Clanging ☐ Echolalia

☐ Incoherent ☐ Neologisms

☐ Receptive Language ☒ Normal ☐ Abnormal

MOOD

☐ Normal ☐ Euphoric ☐ Elevated ☐ Depressed

☐ Angry ☐ Irritable ☒ Anxious

AFFECT

☒ Broad ☐ Restricted ☐ Blunted ☐ Flat

☐ Inappropriate ☐ Labile

ORIENTATION

☒ Normal	☐ Person	☐ Place	☐ Time

ESTIMATED IQ

☐ Above Average	☒ Normal	☐ Below Average

ATTENTION	☒ Normal	☐ Distractible	☐ Hypervigilant
CONCENTRATION	☒ Normal	☐ Brief	

MEMORY

Recent Memory:	☒ Normal	☐ Abnormal
Remote Memory:	☒ Normal	☐ Abnormal

THOUGHT PROCESSES

☒ Normal	☐ Flights of Ideas	☐ Loose	☐ Confabulation
☐ Ideas of Reference	☐ Grandiosity	☐ Paranoia	☐ Magical Thinking
☐ Obsessions	☐ Preservation	☐ Delusions	☐ Depersonalization

Suicidal Ideation None reported

Plan, if so what? None reported

Intent None reported

Previous attempts. If so, was hospitalization required? ☐ Yes ☒ No

Family history of suicide. Who? None reported

Homicidal Ideation. Who? None reported

Plan. If so, what? None reported

Intent None reported

SUBSTANCE ABUSE

Is there any current substance abuse? ☐ Yes ☒ No

If yes, what? ________________ how long? ____________________

Any history of substance abuse? ☐ Yes ☒ No

If yes, what? ________________ when? ____________________ how long? ________

Any family history of substance abuse? ☐ Yes ☒ No If yes, who? ______________

HALLUCINATION

☒ None ☐ Auditory ☐ Visual ☐ Olfactory

JUDGMENT

☐ Good ☐ Fair ☒ Poor

INSIGHT

☒ Good ☐ Fair ☐ Poor

IMPULSE CONTROL

☒ Good ☐ Fair ☐ Poor

ADDITIONAL COMMENTS ____

____

Clinician ____Tara Pist, MEd __________ Date ____3/26/2024________________________

THE CASE OF SUSAN (ENTIRE CASE IN CHAPTER 2)

Susan Thomas is a 43-year-old single mother of three children under age 10. She is currently enrolled in a clinical mental health counseling program at a midsize Midwestern college. Susan's decision to pursue a counseling degree stemmed from a personal tragedy: Her husband passed away 3 years ago due to an accidental drug overdose. Motivated by this experience, Susan embarked on a path to become a substance abuse counselor, aiming to help others navigate similar challenges.

Susan has recently begun experiencing significant stress related to her coursework, specifically during exams and presentations. While she did well in her undergrad psychology program, it was so long ago, and Susan feels that she is not as knowledgeable and skilled with the technical aspects that are required. She often feels behind in her studies and she has to stay up late and work harder than other students in order to feel caught up. Susan feels like she has to spend all of her non-work time on schoolwork, which has become increasingly challenging both emotionally and academically. There are times when it becomes almost impossible to focus, especially when the readings and assignments make her feel that maybe there was more that she could have done to help her husband.

Susan also feels increasingly overwhelmed by the demands of balancing her responsibilities as a mother and a graduate student. Susan's anxiety has started affecting her sleep, appetite, and overall well-being, leading her to seek individual counseling support.

Initial Assessment

In the initial session, Susan shows up 10 minutes early and is eager to begin counseling. Susan shares her background story with many details and cries openly at various times during the session. Susan looks to you for guidance about how she should be feeling. Susan shares current challenges in pursuing her counseling degree. She expresses feeling overwhelmed by academic stress, imposter syndrome, and the demands of parenthood. Susan's grief over her husband's death also emerges as a significant emotional burden.

Susan states that she was living in a small town and moved to a larger city in her state in order to be closer to family and resources for her children. While Susan indicates that she was never close to her mother, she thought that moving closer would strengthen their relationship and that her mother would be able to help with childcare while Susan was busy with work and school. During the intake Susan also details current stressors, including lack of consistent childcare and feeling empty and alone. Susan expresses a strong desire to succeed in her program but feels unsure about managing the academic workload; she has begun to feel imposter syndrome, including thoughts of worthlessness. Though Susan often has thoughts of "Who am I to think that I can help anyone?" she also believes that she needs to "do this" in order to feel good about herself and tells herself, "I am doing this for you [her husband]."

MENTAL STATUS EXAM

Client's Name: Susan Woods **DOB:** 10/24/1980

APPEARANCE

Grooming: ☒ Normal ☐ Disheveled ☐ Unusual

Hygiene: ☒ Normal ☐ Body Odor ☐ Bad Breath ☐ Other________________

MOTOR ACTIVITY

☐ Relaxed ☒ Restless ☐ Pacing ☐ Sedate

☐ Threatening ☐ Catatonic ☐ Posturing ☐ Mannerisms

☐ Tremors ☐ Tics ☐ Psychomotor Retardation

Other ____

INTERPERSONAL

☒ Cooperative ☐ Oppositional/Resistant

☐ Defensive ☐ Other ____________

SPEECH

Characteristics ☒ Normal ☐ Slow ☐ Dysarthric ☐ Apraxic ☐ Pressured

Expressive Language ☒ Normal ☐ Circumstantial ☐ Anomia ☐ Paraphasia ☐ Clanging ☐ Echolalia ☐ Incoherent ☐ Neologisms

Receptive Language ☒ Normal ☐ Abnormal

MOOD

☐ Normal ☐ Euphoric ☐ Elevated ☐ Depressed

☐ Angry ☐ Irritable ☒ Anxious

AFFECT

☒ Broad ☐ Restricted ☐ Blunted ☐ Flat

☐ Inappropriate ☐ Labile

ORIENTATION

☒ Normal ☐ Person ☐ Place ☐ Time

ESTIMATED IQ

Above Average ☒ Normal ☐ Below Average

ATTENTION ☒ Normal ☐ Distractible ☐ Hypervigilant

CONCENTRATION ☒ Normal ☐ Brief

MEMORY

Recent Memory: ☒ Normal ☐ Abnormal

Remote Memory: ☒ Normal ☐ Abnormal

THOUGHT PROCESSES

☒ Normal	☐ Flights of Ideas	☐ Loose	☐ Confabulation
☐ Ideas of Reference	☐ Grandiosity	☐ Paranoia	☐ Magical Thinking
☐ Obsessions	☐ Preservation	☐ Delusions	☐ Depersonalization

Suicidal Ideation None reported

Plan. If so, what? None reported

Intent None reported

Previous attempts. If so, was hospitalization required? ☐ Yes ☒ No

Family history of suicide. Who? None reported

Homicidal ideation. Who? None reported

Plan. If so, what? None reported

Intent None reported

SUBSTANCE ABUSE

Is there any current substance abuse/misuse? ☐ Yes ☒ No

If yes, what? ____________ how long? ___________

Any history of substance abuse? ☐ Yes ☒ No

If yes, what? ____________ when? __________ how long? _________

Any family history of substance abuse? ☒ Yes ☐ No

If yes, who? Husband died of drug overdose

HALLUCINATION

☒ None ☐ Auditory ☐ Visual ☐ Olfactory

JUDGMENT

☐ Good ☒ Fair ☐ Poor

INSIGHT

☒ Good ☐ Fair ☐ Poor

IMPULSE CONTROL

☒ Good ☐ Fair ☐ Poor

ADDITIONAL COMMENTS ____________________

____

Clinician ______Gene Hudlow, MEd, LPCC______ Date ______6/14/2024______

REFERENCES

American Counseling Association. (2014). *2014 ACA code of ethics.* https://www.counseling.org/docs/

American Psychiatric Association. (2022). *Diagnostic and statistical manual of mental disorders* (5th ed., text rev.).

American Psychological Association. (2017). *Ethical principles of psychologists and code of conduct.* https://www.apa.org/ethics/code

Baird, B. (2005). *The internship, practicum, and field placement handbook: A guide for the helping professions (4th ed.).* Routledge.

Capuzzi, D., & Stauffer, M. D. (2020). *Foundations for addiction counseling (4th ed.).* Pearson.

Carlson, J. F. (2016). Clinical assessment. In H. S. Friedman (Ed.), *Encyclopedia of mental health* (2nd ed., pp. 293–297). Elsevier. https://www.sciencedirect.com/referencework/9780123977533/encyclopedia-of-mental-health

Gehart, D. (2016). *Case documentation in counseling and psychotherapy: A theory-informed, competency-based approach.* Cengage Learning.

Gill, C. S., Harper, M. C., & Dailey, S. F. (2014). Assessing the spiritual and religious domain. In C. S. Cashwell & J. S. Young (Eds.), *Integrating religion and spirituality in counseling: A guide to competent practice* (2nd ed., pp. 141–162). American Counseling Association.

Griffin, M. (2022, July 5). *Attorney articles: Ethical considerations in treatment planning.* California Association of Marriage and Family Therapists. https://www.camft.org/

Healthcare Providers Service Organization. (2019, March). *Counselor liability claim report (2nd ed.).* https://www.hpso.com/getmedia/ac13a1d8-3bdd-4117-ad36-8fba7c419153/counselor-claim-report-second-edition.pdf

Ivey, A. E., Ivey, M. B., & Zalaquett, C. P. (2018). *Intentional interviewing and counseling: Facilitating client development in a multicultural society* (9th ed.). Cengage Learning.

Johnson, S. L. (2018). *Therapist's guide to clinical intervention: The 1-2-3's of treatment planning* (3rd ed.). Academic Press.

Jull, G., Sterling, M., Falla, D., Treleaven, J., & O'Leary, S. (2008). *Whiplash, headache, and neck pain: Research-based directions for physical therapies.* https://www.sciencedirect.com/book/9780443100475/whiplash-headache-and-neck-pain

National Association of Social Workers. (2021). *Code of ethics of the National Association of Social Workers.* https://www.socialworkers.org/About/Ethics/Code-of-Ethics/Code-of-Ethics

Nishioka, S., Hunt, E., & Snyder, S. E. (2023). Assessment, clinical formulation, and diagnosis: A biopsychosocial framework within the developmental systems lens. In S. Snyder (Ed.), *A developmental systems guide for child and adolescent behavioral health practitioners.* Temple University Press. https://temple.manifoldapp.org/read/a-developmental_systems-guide-for-child-and-adolescent-behavioral-health-practitioners-da7c780a=719d-4c6a-ad85-b6736f8df14f/section/

Oregon Health Care Association. (2017, March 2). Article 10: Clinical assessment. *Carenotes.* https://www.ohca.com/carenotes

Piazza, N. J., & Baruth, N. E. (1990). Client record guidelines. *Journal of Counseling & Development, 68,* 313–316.

Sheparis, C. J., Drummond, R. J., & Jones, K. D. (2020). *Assessment procedures for counselors and helping professionals* (9th ed.). Pearson.

Voss, R. M., & M Das, J. (2022). *Mental Status Examination*. StatPearls. https://www.ncbi.nlm.nih.gov/books/NBK546682/

Weiner, I. B. (2004) Clinical assessment. In C. Spielberger (Ed.), *Encyclopedia of applied psychology (1st ed.*, pp. 351–355). Elsevier. https://www.sciencedirect.com/science/article/abs/pii/B0126574103005134

Whiston, S. C. (2017). *Principles and applications of assessment in counseling* (5th ed.). Cengage Learning.

CHAPTER 6

Case Conceptualization

Mona Gallo, EdD, Melinda Mays, EdD, Gregory L. Bohner, PhD, Daniel R. Romero, PhD, and Holly J. Mattingly, PhD

INTRODUCTION

Generally, following obtaining an informed consent, any releases of information, and a mental health intake and/or assessment with clients, clinicians will begin the process of developing a case conceptualization (CC), sometimes referred to as a *case formulation* (Osborn et al., 2004; Prieto & Scheel, 2002). The method of conceptualizing a case is when a clinician acquires and organizes the client's clinical information. The development and use of a CC is the key piece of documentation that represents the client's clinical presentation, like a snapshot in time, yet the CC is not necessarily a static document. Documenting the CC may be an ongoing process (Easden & Kazantzis, 2016; Osborn et al., 2004), may evolve across the client's treatment, and may only conclude at the client's discharge. The ongoing process can occur because the client's treatment is generally not stagnant, as clients are participants in their life and treatment. The client may glean more clarity as they move further away from their problem, the client remembers more details, stakeholders contribute additional information, and the clinician's interpretations become clearer through clinical contact. If the CC needs to be added to or changed, the clinician can create an addendum that includes the new or updated data, or the clinician can draft an entirely new CC document with the previous and more current data.

Given the magnitude of clinical data collected, developing and documenting a CC can sometimes seem like an overwhelming task, and some clinicians may dismiss this process in favor of just relying on a diagnosis to manage large client caseloads (Osborn et al., 2004). Clinicians in training are frequently taught the skill of developing a CC to help the trainee evaluate and consider how all the client information gained in a few initial sessions can lend itself to a diagnosis, an appropriate theory to use with the client, and the development of a course for treatment through the development of a treatment plan (Sperry, 2005a).

It is important that a clinician is trained in developing and utilizing a client CC because it informs treatment decisions more thoroughly, considering the client's specific characteristics and unique situations that diagnosis alone may not delineate (Groenier et al., 2014), and it is a foundational skill in the development of effective treatment planning and more positive treatment outcomes (Sperry, 2005b). Being able to conceptualize client cases is a skill that is gained through educational training and instruction, supervision, and repeated application (Prieto & Scheel, 2002; Sperry, 2005b). Effective clinicians can draw out client information to develop and generate CCs and recognize the value in the development of a CC to steer the development of a treatment plan and guide the client's treatment (Sperry, 2005a).

ETHICAL NEED FOR DOCUMENTING IN CASE CONCEPTUALIZATION

A case conceptualization can be the foundational piece of documentation that demonstrates the basis for decisions regarding treatment, as well as monitoring and evaluating treatment efficacy (Osborn et al., 2004; Sperry, 2005a). While a CC document may not be required as part of a client's formal record, as the intake and assessment may be, a clinician's ability to postulate a theory or idea of what may be going on with their client is of utmost importance. Because of this, clinicians in training require an abundance of clinical supervision and discussion surrounding their specific clients and details, all of which are significant for best treatment interventions. The conceptualization of a client case and story includes information from clinical observation, intake and assessment material, as well as possibly collateral information from third parties (e.g., parents and family members, teachers, other mental health and medical professionals, etc.). Because of the complexity and uniqueness of individual clients, a clinician must always be open and prepared to consider new and/or changing information to develop and grow their conceptualization for the best ethical treatment.

While no literature addresses specific ethical codes related to conceptualizing client cases, it is of the utmost importance to follow the ethical guidelines regarding confidentiality, record storage and transfer, as well as client access to records. It is also important to consider that ethically, it is important to identify and utilize the client's diversity within their situations, relationships, and problems. However, the balance is that the clinician does not focus so intently on diversity that they miss imperative clinical considerations (Neufeldt et al., 2006).

LEGAL NEED FOR DOCUMENTING IN CASE CONCEPTUALIZATION

A case conceptualization can demonstrate a clinician's diagnostic capacity, clinical thinking and judgment, and treatment considerations for best client care. A well-documented CC can also aid a clinician in the event there is a legal or license board query. Since there are many details that are synthesized and documented in a CC, it is crucial for clinicians to consider meticulously documenting all relevant details within the client's CC. According to the Healthcare Providers Service Organization (2019), the strongest defense for a clinician is when the clinician has comprehensively documented their decision-making process, the client's diagnosis, the treatment plan, the education of the client to the treatment plan and policies related to treatment, the client's responses to treatment, diagnostic testing and the results, assessment of the client's risk and the results of the assessment, referrals for medical assessment, prescriptions used and who is monitoring the client while they are using psychotropic medication, any materials provided to the client for educational or resource purposes, the client's participation in treatment, and referrals. Ultimately, the CC can synthesis all this data and should reflect the clinician's support of a plan for the client's treatment.

A review of the literature regarding specific laws and regulations related to case conceptualization did not yield specific mandates; however, there are federal regulations (National Archives, 2013) that require the clinician to have a full and complete understanding of the client's strengths, weaknesses, resilience, and functioning which is determined through clinical interviews and diagnostic assessments and often reported in a case conceptualization. Related guidelines noted by many states' licensing boards require case conceptualization training to be included in the curriculum of counseling, social work, and psychology programs.

THE PURPOSE OF DEVELOPING A CASE CONCEPTUALIZATION

The purpose of developing a case conceptualization is for the clinician to document and analyze the client's data, formulate clinical judgments, and then to consider the purpose and implement treatment decisions (Falvey, 2001; Osborn et al., 2004). Both the clinical and treatment formulation portions of the client's case require the clinician to use deductive and inductive reasoning (Sperry, 2005b). Both types of reasoning can lead clinicians to more comprehensive CCs and better client treatment. *Deductive reasoning* is a logical approach to progress from general ideas to more precise conclusions. An example of deductive reasoning is "Point A data leads to Point B conclusion." *Inductive reasoning*, on the other hand, is more of a logical progression that includes multiple ideas that can be a combination of experiences, observations, and facts, which are then combined to develop more exact conclusions. An example of inductive reasoning is "Points A, E, K, and M data lead to Point B conclusion."

The CC is more than a written document that the clinician refers or adds to, as it is integral to the clinician's dynamic clinical knowledge of the client, the clinical landscape through which the clinician views, understands, and ultimately treats and helps the client. The CC is, in a sense, the operationalization of all the gathered client information that the clinician uses to frame and guide their work with the client. This document serves as a summary of the client's current and historical data provided by the client and stakeholders (Gazzillo et al., 2021; Lenz & Litam, 2023; Sperry, 2005a). The data in the CC accounts for the client's operative relationship between their experiences and mental health. It encompasses the meaning of a client's problems and symptoms and hypothesizes the explanation of client choices and behaviors (Sperry, 2005a).

Another purpose in developing a CC is that the collected data is compiled in one place that will guide the clinician in the client's treatment. The CC outlines the client's treatment direction and process through proposed treatment direction through individual and system strategies, interventions, and plans for prevention (Hagmayer et al., 2021; Lenz & Litam, 2023). This document aids clinicians and clients in maintaining a treatment direction, which has been shown to contribute to positive treatment outcomes (Maniacci et al., 2017). Through a clinician's clinical and theoretical interpretations expressed in a CC, the client's hypothetical future is a comprehensive depiction of what the client is attempting to attain from treatment, any obstacles that may prevent the attainment of the client's goals, and the client's willingness to pursue achieving their goals (Gazzillo et al., 2021; Hagmayer et al., 2021; Sperry, 2005a).

Additionally, using a CC can aid a clinician in informing the client about the complexity of their difficulties and can support the clinician and client in evaluating the impact of the client's circumstances and can provide a roadmap to recovery from mental health concerns (Hagmayer et al., 2021; Lenz & Litam, 2023; Maniacci et al., 2017; Sperry, 2017). When a clinician utilizes a CC with a client, the client becomes a collaborative participant in their own treatment and can more clearly work toward achieving their own goals. The client's participation in the development of the CC is to describe their concerns, their symptoms (and rate their perception of their impairment), and their goals, as well as expectations of treatment. This offers the opportunity for the clinician not only to view the client from a clinical lens but also to hear and consider the client's view and input on the CC and treatment plan (see Chapter 7). The client's collaboration in their treatment has been shown to be more supportive in the client's engagement and commitment to their treatment (Sperry, 2005a).

Another purpose in developing a CC is that it may be required by clinics, agencies, and third-party payers to demonstrate evidence-based treatment compliance. A CC can not only provide valuable information to other providers involved in the client's treatment but also guide a clinician during client case review during treatment team meetings.

Lastly, a CC can be used during supervision to guide case discussion and case-specific details. Supervisors may also utilize the CC as a means of monitoring a supervisee's development with specific client cases (Prieto & Scheel, 2002; Sperry, 2005a).

TYPES OF CASE CONCEPTUALIZATION

According to Sperry (2005a), there are three types of case conceptualizations with different focuses: symptom (diagnostic), theory, or client. A comprehensive CC would contain all three components (Sperry, 2005a; 2005b). Clinicians can use culturally informed CC formats in comprehensive CCs to provide depth and breath in the development of their CCs. One such culturally informed CC format is ADDRESSING—an acronym for age, developmental and acquired disabilities, religion, ethnicity, socioeconomic status, sexual orientation, indigenous heritage, national origin, and gender (Lake et al., 2022). It is important to include cultural information in the client's CC, but only utilizing a culturally informed format is not considered thorough enough for treatment purposes.

Clinically Focused Case Conceptualization

The diagnostic component is meant to aid the clinician in developing a clinical formulation. Developing a comprehensive CC illustrates the clinician's understanding of the client's symptomatology and the context in which they appeared and are being perpetuated. It is the foundation for a successful treatment plan and client prognosis (Lenz & Litam, 2023; Osborn et al., 2004).

Documenting the clinical data is only the beginning of a clinically focused CC because complex clinical data without a clinical interpretation does not necessarily provide a treatment direction or adequate treatment interventions (Falvey, 2001). The clinical interpretations are founded on a combination of the unique client data presented and the clinician's lens that considers the underlying influencing factors that may be contributing to the client's presentation (Lenz & Litam, 2023). The interpretations of the clinical data include the clinician's perceptions of the client's situation, analysis of any maladaptive patterns, as well as charting the focus of treatment while considering any potential difficulties or barriers to the client successfully obtaining the goals and ultimately the successful termination of therapy (Sperry & Sperry, 2020).

Theory-Focused Case Conceptualization

The use of the clinician's theoretical view of treatment generally first appears in writing within the CC. The use of a theoretical lens can assist clinicians in providing a foundation of explanation for the client's symptoms and behaviors (Groenier et al., 2014; Sperry, 2005b) and can link the data collected from the client and the clinical observations into one comprehensive clinical document (Sperry, 2005b). The use of a theoretical lens also assists the clinician in developing a treatment direction through goal setting and by therapeutic interventions (see Chapter 7). The development of theoretically driven treatment goals and interventions may not only relieve the client's symptoms but also provide a framework of understanding to the client as to reasons they may have developed dysfunctional behaviors. By developing a view of the client's symptoms, behaviors, treatment direction, and interventions through a theoretical lens, the clinician may have an increased ability to understand the client's relational, cultural, and systemic orientation and how the interplay of the client in context may be supporting or exasperating the client's symptoms and behaviors (Osborn et al., 2004; Sperry, 2005a).

There are various theoretical models and theory-specific approaches that can inform the development of the CC. Hagmayer et al. (2021) emphasizes that the model chosen "has to be based on empirically validated theoretical models of psychopathology" (p. 649). An in-depth summary of the presented options is beyond the scope of this book, and only a sampling and a brief overview of what is available is provided.

The 5Ps approach offers a framework for the clinician to evaluate and document the presenting problem, predisposing factors, precipitating factors, perpetuating factors, and the protective/positive factors (Macneil et al., 2012). The client map offers a visual representation of counseling and the decision-making process for the clinician and client to enhance communications (Lenz & Litam, 2023). There are cognitive behavioral approaches that emphasize the use of CC to support the clinician's understanding of the client's etiology and maintenance of their problems and is central in the establishment of relevant interventions (Easden & Kazantzis, 2016). Disorder-specific models are utilized when the client presents with a single diagnosis and treatment addressing alleviating or eliminating the symptomology, whereas the transdiagnostic model would address co- or multi-morbidity. The PACT model is one such transdiagnostic model that addresses the protocol for assessment, case formulation, and treatment planning functions of treatment (Hagmayer et al., 2021). Clinicians can find CC formats from specific theoretical approaches, such as Adlerian (Sperry, 2017), cognitive behavioral (Beck, 1995; Cronin et al., 2015), and others.

One limitation in using a theoretical lens to view the client's problems in a CC is that the theoretical lens may only speak to the clinician. A theoretical view is clinician-centered, and this perspective may not be reflective of how the client may perceive their own problems. If the client cannot conceptualize their own problems through the clinician's theoretical lens, then the client's commitment to the treatment direction, goals, and interventions may become limited and treatment may stall or be prematurely terminated (Sperry, 2005a).

Client-Focused Case Conceptualization

A client-focused CC is developed from the client's perspective—their needs and their expectations. The clinician would comprehensively listen to the client's presenting problems, immerse themselves in the client's understanding of relational concerns, and consider cultural or systemic factors of the client prior to choosing a theoretical approach in their work with the client. A client-focused CC may maximize a match between the client problems and symptoms, goals and interventions, and potentially lead to better treatment outcomes and more of a commitment from the client to their treatment (Sperry, 2005).

THE DATA CONTAINED WITHIN A CASE CONCEPTUALIZATION

The more client data the clinician can collect, the better the opportunity for the clinician to conceptualize the client's case more accurately. However, the more clinical data the clinician has, the more difficult the case may be to conceptualize, which can potentially lead to the clinician's lack of confidence in conceptualizing a client's case (Falvey, 2001; Sperry, 2005b). A thorough CC will include at least these basic elements: a description of the client's presenting problem(s), their developmental history, the clinician's evidence-based interpretations regarding the factors that cause or maintain the client's past and/or current functioning, any strengths or weaknesses in coping, and the recommendations for treatment (Groenier et al., 2014).

CCs can take many forms. Utilizing a CC template or format may assist clinicians in more clearly conceptualizing the client's case. Often, places of service will have a template or format that is offered to assist clinicians in completing this foundational treatment data. If a treatment facility lacks a required or recommended format, the following information can aid clinicians in developing a comprehensive CC. Suggested portions of a comprehensive CC include the client's presenting problems and considers the client's biological, psychological, environmental, social-cultural, developmental, and etiological domains. Some agencies desire clinicians to add client identifying information, which may include any or all the following: date of birth, contact information, Social Security number, marital status, children, occupation, educational level, income, cultural identity, medical history, current medication, history or current substance abuse/misuse, and legal history. Most frameworks of a CC also include family-of-origin data such as composition of the family of origin, history of mental or emotional disorders, and any substance abuse/misuse history. Clinical data that has been obtained through client statements needs to clearly reflect that the data has been reported, such as "The client reported ..." or "The client stated. ..."

The clinician may include observational data such as the client's appearance at appointments, their interpersonal interaction with the clinician or staff, the client's cognitive, emotional, and behavioral factors, the client's current social and psychological resources, and the client's current coping skills and strengths. Clinical data would include symptoms of distress or impaired functioning, a diagnosis or provisional diagnosis, any differential diagnoses, and a diagnostic rationale. The clinician would also include their understanding of how the use of theory can aid the client, the client's impairment of functioning, the client's prognosis, the nature of treatment (i.e., group, individual, case management, etc.), and any potential referrals. When documenting clinical data obtained from observation of the client, use phrases such as "The clinician observed ..." "It seemed ... by evidence of ..." or "It appears the client ... by evidence of. ..."

A problematic area that may often get overlooked by clinicians developing a CC is the consideration of biological or physiological implications related to the client's problems. Gathering as much medical data as possible is imperative in thoroughly hypothesizing the client's case (Cipani & Golden, 2007). For example, a child may have been a rather pleasant and cooperative child until just a few months ago. Without a complete understanding of any invisible physiological occurrences, a clinician may mistakenly suspect a change in the child's environment, some occurrence regarding trauma, or changes in interpersonal relationships. In a case where a change in a client's presentation is dramatic, it is critical that a clinician consider a referral to a medical professional to investigate any physiological change before diagnosing and developing a clinical and treatment formulation for the case.

Another problematic area in developing a CC is that the clinician's theoretical lens may influence the clinicians to unduly focus too closely on one area (i.e., diagnostic, clinical, client) over another. The data in the CC needs to be as detailed as possible, considering all the data collected and not minimizing details that can inform the clinician's clinical formation of the client's case, which ultimately can influence the treatment direction. It is imperative for clinicians to consider all data to develop a well-informed and well-documented CC and not overlook any environmental or interpersonal influences that may be precipitating the client's symptoms, behaviors, or choices (Cipani & Golden, 2007). Examples of times a clinician may unduly exclude critical data would include (a) a behavioral-centered clinician not considering the environmental influence as deeply as a systems-centered clinician or (b) a person-centered clinician not considering the client's family-of-origin complexities as deeply as an Adlerian-centered clinician.

The CC includes data related to the client's inner world, how they operate interpersonally, as well as within the context of their systems (e.g., work, family, neighborhood, etc.). The clinician may also include the cause of the client's symptoms or life patterns from data the client reports or the clinician's interpretation (Lenz & Litam, 2023).

Physiological Data

The *physiological data* consists of the physiological and genetic components and how they may be contributing to the client's mental health. This includes organic functions, the genetic predisposition, the functioning of immune and hormonal systems, and neurological status. These physiological factors may be affected by internal and external variables and may influence one another in either or both directions (Lenz & Litam, 2023). Regulating the client's physiology and biology through medication interventions should be left to the adjunct medical provider with full consent, participation, and cooperation from the client and should involve keeping the clinician informed on this process and decisions.

Psychological Data

The *psychological data* consists of "the cognitive, emotional, motivational, attitudinal, and behavioral systems that affect and cause mental health and illness" (Lenz & Litam, 2023, p. 420). Clinicians would observe the client's patterns through the client's cognitive, emotional, and personality characteristics; attitudes; personal beliefs about the self, others, and world at large, as well as the ability to cope with their experiences (Lenz & Litam, 2023). The client's psychological presentation may have protective and risk factors. These psychological factors may also be affected by internal and external variables and may influence one another in either or both directions.

Environmental Data

Environmental data includes all the pertinent information about the client's living situation within the context of their systems. This would include information about the client's work, family, neighborhood, community, socioeconomic status, living situation, and any other pertinent information that might shed light on the client's level of functioning (Lenz & Litam, 2023). There are several ways that the information from the environment can be critical in making an accurate conceptualization of the client. Analysis of the environment may help identify, define, and clarify environmental opportunities and supports (Hurst & McKinley, 1988). The environment also will likely have factors that might either trigger or reinforce certain behaviors. Exploration of the environment will also help the clinician discover any challenges or negative influences that may affect the client's prognosis.

Sociocultural Data

The *sociocultural data* includes the client's perception of or factual elements of the social and cultural context in which the client may have direct or indirect contact and influence from others (Lehman et al., 2017). The client's interpersonal interactions have an influence on the client's mental health, feelings of safety and belonging, and opportunities for positive outcomes. Additional sociocultural data that clinicians may collect from client interactions are ones related to the political climate, regulations and policies, and any social norms that may influence the client's community (Lenz & Litam, 2023). These factors can span across the client's life or be isolated to a specific place, time, age, and so on. Not all clients will be affected by sociocultural factors, but an astute clinician can observe, clarify, and hypothesize how these factors may be contributing to the client's resiliency or may be underlying a mental health condition.

Developmental Data

The *developmental data* includes information that may reflect the genetic and biological components related to the client's experiences across their sections of lifetime development (Sperry, 2005a). The "developmental experiences that influence mental health are neither static nor linear, but instead dynamic, multidirectional, and multideterminate" (Lenz & Litam, 2023, p. 421). Therefore, the developmental data may reflect etiological, maintenance, and/or mitigating factors.

Etiology is when there is some type of cause or influence. Related to mental health, the *etiological factors* can be identified as the origin of the client symptoms and potential impairment. They would have a primary role in forming the development and welfare of the client's symptomology because of their heritability and influence on a mental health condition and the effect on the client. Etiological factors are not limited to only biological or physiological sources. Clinicians need to be aware that etiological factors may span across biopsychosocial-cultural domains and consider a wider lens in viewing the client's presentation from a perspective of how they as an individual have engaged with and been impacted by the environment across time (Lenz & Litam, 2023; Macneil et al., 2012; Osborn et al., 2004).

Maintenance factors are the experiences that the client has or is involved in that may stem from circumstances, events, or activities. These factors would have a direct positive or negative impact on the client's mental health. Maintenance factors are the client's cognitive, behavioral, emotional, environmental, and/or interpersonal components that may be perpetuating their symptomatology, as well as the severity and impairment. The level to which these maintenance factors are either adaptive or maladaptive is relative to the client's perspective of their functionality. If the maintenance factors are productive, then the client will be or has been influenced positively. If not, the client will have developed maladaptive patterns and be limited in their adaptation and growth. Clinicians can assist their clients in identifying these maintenance factors and use this data to influence the client's treatment objectives and interventions (Groenier et al., 2014; Hagmayer et al., 2021; Lenz & Litam, 2023; Osborn et al., 2004).

Mitigating factors are developed from the clinician and client's identification and logical connection between the etiological and maintenance factors. Mitigating factors in treatment may appear as any support, education, and interventions that assist the reduction of the client's symptomatology, serve as a protective factor, and may prevent additional risk. Clinicians need to consider that the mitigating factors need to be culturally congruent for the client, informed by theory, and accessible to the client (Lenz & Litam, 2023).

Diagnostic Portion of Case Conceptualization

Diagnosis is an essential part of mental health treatment; and often, treatment is not reimbursable without it. Generally, the first time a diagnosis, provisional diagnosis, and differential diagnosis(es) emerges is in a CC. A well-thought-out and comprehensively developed CC that considers all data aids clinicians in developing a deeper diagnostic, clinical, and treatment formulation of a client's case. This process supports clinicians with a rationale and structure to deliver appropriate objectives, activities, interventions, education, referrals, and potentially a more successful course of treatment (Lenz & Litam, 2023).

The diagnostic portion of the CC focuses on the client's symptoms and impairment and is frequently supported using the current edition of the American Psychiatric Association's *Diagnostic and Statistical Manual of Mental Disorders* (currently the *DSM-5-TR*). Within the CC, the diagnosis is supported by descriptive statements that include the nature and severity of the client's presentation (Sperry, 2005a; 2005b). Sperry (2005a) stresses that "diagnostic formulations are descriptive, phenomenological, and cross-sectional in nature" (p. 190), and the diagnostic formulation assists the clinician in developing a diagnostic conclusion. In part, this portion of the CC informs the development of measurable goals, objectives, and interventions targeted at reducing the client's symptoms and improving functionality. Symptom-focused treatment aids in accountability because the goals and objectives are generally easier to monitor and measure (Groenier et al., 2014; Sperry, 2005a; 2005b).

There can be some concerns regarding diagnosing a client immediately following an intake or just after a few sessions, which is often what is required in completing a CC. Sometimes it may be difficult to diagnose a client so rapidly. Other times, a client arrives with a previous diagnosis that the clinician would need to verify and confirm. And there are times the client has an array of symptoms that do not lead to one distinct diagnosis, at least initially. In this case, a provisional diagnosis is not just appropriate but warranted.

Clinicians are cautioned not to use common mental shortcuts to simplify diagnostic uncertainty. Although a heuristic diagnostic process can be a time-saver, it can be fraught with problems. A clinician could mistakenly attribute symptoms to an incorrect diagnosis, could potentially seek out information from the client or stakeholders that could create a confirmation bias, or overly simplify the process of gathering information leading to a hasty conclusion regarding diagnosis or treatment. Other mental shortcut errors that can potentially occur are recalling case information that may be from a different case, potentially imposing personal beliefs when objective information is unavailable, and quickly deducing conclusions with very little data presented (Falvey et al., 2005).

It is essential that the clinician includes more than simple diagnosis in a CC. Crucial components that justify a mental health diagnosis include information regarding the client's symptoms, specifiers, length and duration of impairment, the elimination of other potential causes, the context of the client's symptoms, the history of the client's problems, accurate details from assessment data, and the clinician's judgment (Falvey, 2001; Lenz & Litam, 2023). It is imperative that the clinician understands the context, risk factors, and protective variables that influence the persistence of symptoms and alleviation of them (Lenz & Litam, 2023). Gaining the correct case history and diagnostic information is essential in the development of the clinician's clinical formulation of the case (Falvey, 2001). But if the clinician only focuses on the diagnostic portion of a CC, then treatment can miss the benefit of a clinical formulation of the client's problems (Groenier et al., 2014).

CONCLUSION

A comprehensive CC can support the clinician in developing a road map for the client's treatment (Osborn et al., 2004). The CC is a long-range perspective that includes objective data and the clinician's interpretation regarding the client's establishment and perpetuation of the client's "symptoms and dysfunctional life patterns ... [as well as, the client's] ... predictable style of thinking, feeling, acting, and coping in stressful circumstances" (Sperry, 2005a, p. 190). The data collected and clinical formulation will retain details, depict the influence and interconnectedness of the data across time, and represent the collaborative nature of treatment (Lenz & Litam, 2023).

Together, the diagnostic and clinical formulation can provide a solid foundation for the clinician and client to develop a clearer course of treatment. The treatment formulation, addressed thoroughly in Chapter 7, is comprised of clear problems, well-articulated goals to resolve the problems, objectives that are the small steps the client agrees to take to attain the overall goal, the treatment interventions that will be utilized for the client to achieve the objectives, as well as any clinical prognosis regarding treatment outcomes (Sperry, 2005a, 2005b).

EXAMPLE CASE CONCEPTUALIZATION FORMAT

Client Demographic Data

1. Name (initials or altered name for confidentiality)
2. Date of birth/age
3. Sex
4. Marital status
5. Children (in and out of home, ages, sex)
6. Living situation (house or apartment, people living in the home and relationship with client)

Socioeconomic Status Data

1. Occupation status
2. Client income, education
3. Family members' education
4. Average family income
5. Transportation status (drives own car, public transportation)
6. Other economic resources (own house, savings, family support)
7. Economic stressors (debts, child support, etc.)

Presenting Problem(s): Include a description of the problem areas, listed separately, from the client's perspective, particularly noting client's view of their order of importance. Suggested items of focus:

1. Were there precipitating factors?
2. How long have the problems persisted?
3. Have problems previously occurred? What were the circumstances?
4. In what way, if any, do the problems relate to each other?
5. Presence of suicide risk or ideation?

Relevant History

This section will vary in comprehension according to depth and length of treatment and in focus according to theoretical orientation and specific nature of problems. Suggested focus:

1. Family and relationship history (family of origin/developmental issues, past)
    - marriages/significant relationships—duration, sexual functioning, dissolution factors, sexual orientation, history and/or presence of domestic abuse, etc.
    - children—from current or prior relationships and current status, current family status and structure
2. Cultural history and identity (issues of ethnicity and race, identification/acculturation)
3. Educational history (childhood/developmental, adulthood/current status)

4. Vocational history (types, stability, satisfaction)
5. Medical history (acute/chronic illness, hospitalizations, surgeries, major patterns of illness in family, accidents, injuries, with whom/where/how often receive medical care, etc.)
6. Health practices (sleeping, eating patterns, use of tobacco, consumption of caffeine, etc.)
7. Mental health history (prior problems, symptoms, diagnoses, evaluations, therapy experiences, past prescribed medications, current and family-of-origin mental health histories)
8. Current medications (dosages, purposes, physician, compliance, effects, side effects, etc.)
9. Legal history (arrests, DUI, jail/prison, lawsuits, any pending legal actions)
10. Use/abuse of alcohol or drugs (prescription or illegal)
11. Family (current and origin) alcohol/drug history

Interpersonal Factors

This section contains a description of client's orientation toward others in environment.

1. Manner of dress
2. Physical appearance
3. General self-presentation
4. Nature of typical relationship (dependent, submissive, aggressive, dominant, withdrawing, etc.)
5. Behavior toward therapist (therapeutic alliance)

Environmental Factors

1. Elements in the environment, not already mentioned, that function as stressors to the client—those centrally related to the presenting problems and more peripheral
2. Elements in the environment, not previously mentioned, that function as support for client (friends, family, recreational activities, etc.)

Personality Dynamics

1. Cognitive factors: data related to thinking and mental processes such as intelligence, mental alertness, persistence of negative cognitions, positive cognitions, nature and content of fantasy life, level of insight (awareness of changes in feelings, behavior, reactions of others, understanding of the interplay, etc.), and capacity for judgment (ability to make decisions and carry out practical affairs of daily living)
2. Emotional factors such as typical or most common emotional stress, predominant mood during interviews, appropriateness of affect, range of emotions client can display, cyclical aspects of client's emotional life
3. Behavior factors, such as psychosomatic symptoms and existence of problematic habits or mannerisms

Life Transition/Adaptation Skills

1. Coping skills: concrete efforts to deal with distressing situations (anticipation, preparation, response)
2. Social resources: summary of supportive social networks
3. Psychological resources: adaptive personality characteristics (self-efficacy, hardiness, optimism)

Formal Diagnosis

- ICD-10 Code, Diagnosis, Specifiers—and include at least 1 (one)
- At least 2—ICD-10 Code, Differential Diagnosis

Diagnostic Rationale

- Discussion of symptoms/criteria showing how client meets the diagnostic criteria for the diagnoses given above.
- Include the differential diagnoses, demonstrating you ruled out at least two other diagnoses.

Theoretical Conceptualization of the Case

- First, identify the specific theory or theories used and provide a brief overview of the general theory's main points.
- Next, describe how the conceptualization was then applied to understand the existence of this client's problems.
- Finally, describe how the conceptualization affected the therapist's approach to treatment, which may also include discussion related to multicultural variables.

Recommendations

Each of the following are required to be included in your recommendations:

- Prognosis
- Should services continue to be offered, or would a referral for counseling services elsewhere be more appropriate?
- Potential referral(s) to other professions (e.g., medical, psychiatric, etc.)
- Recommendation for a specific therapeutic orientation to be used with this client
- Nature of treatment (e.g., specific therapist, priority of treatment issues, interaction with client characteristics such as defensiveness, motivation for treatment, problem complexity, etc.)
- Format recommendations concerning working with the client (e.g., individual, group therapy, etc.)

CASE OF ABEL (ENTIRE CASE IN CHAPTER 2)

CASE CONCEPTUALIZATION

Client Demographic Data

1. Abel Tesfaye
2. Age 32, DOB 04/16/1992
3. Male
4. Married
5. 1 child, aged 10. Children all live with client.
6. Client owns his home and lives in the home with his spouse and son.

SES Data

1. Works full time and student
2. Client Income: $42,000/year
3. Education: High school
4. Family members' education: Spouse has a master's degree. Son is currently in elementary school.
5. Average family income: $162,000/year
6. Transportation status: Owns own vehicle
7. Other economic resources: None identified
8. Economic stressors: None identified

Presenting Problem(s):

Client is returning home after hospitalization from suicidal ideation and wants to address his depressive symptoms. In addition, he wants to improve the relationship with his spouse so that it becomes "more bearable."

Relevant History

1. **Family and relationship history**

   Client is a 32-year-old, heterosexual, Black man, married with one child age 10. Client denies history of domestic abuse but describes instances of yelling with spouse with physical intimidation. When asked further, client shrugged and said, "Isn't that how all families fight?" Client identifies his relationship with his mother as a positive one but says that his father has "mean" and "never liked me." Client appears to have a cordial relationship with his mother-in-law.

2. **Cultural history and identity (issues of ethnicity and race, identification/acculturation)**

   Client described concerns related to religious preference, particularly related to his son. He and his spouse have different views on how to raise their son spiritually. He also describes instances of racism he has experienced as a Black man.

3. **Educational history (childhood/developmental, adulthood/current status)**
   Client is currently in school to obtain his associate's degree and plans to pursue a bachelor's degree afterward. No educational or developmental concerns were raised.
4. **Vocational history (types, stability, satisfaction)**
   Client currently works as a truck driver in a factory. He plans on applying for other positions after obtaining his degree in accounting.
5. **Medical history (acute/chronic illness, hospitalizations, surgeries, major patterns of illness in family, accidents, injuries, with whom/where/how often receive medical care, etc.)**
   Client did not disclose any medical concerns or hospitalization for physical conditions.
6. **Health practices (sleeping, eating patterns, use of tobacco, consumption of caffeine, etc.)**
   Client discussed wanting to improve eating patterns with choosing healthier types of food. He also disclosed sleeping problems when he is "in a funk."
7. **Mental health history (prior problems, symptoms, diagnoses, evaluations, therapy experiences, past prescribed medications, current and family-of-origin mental health histories)**
   Client has recently been hospitalized for suicidal ideation. He reports no current ideation, means, or plan.
8. **Current medications (dosages, purposes, physician, compliance, effects, side effects, etc.)**
   Client indicates he is currently taking 60mg once daily. He claims to be compliant and says the side effects have not been severe.
9. **Legal history (arrests, DUI, jail/prison, lawsuits, any pending legal actions)**
   Client denies any arrests, DUIs, or legal history.
10. **Use/misuse of alcohol or drugs (prescription or illegal)**
    Client denies use of alcohol or drugs.
11. **Family (current and origin) alcohol/drug history**
    Client denies any family history of drug or alcohol use or misuse.

Interpersonal Factors

This section contains a description of the client's orientation toward others in the environment.

1. **Manner of dress**
   Client dressed in his work uniform. His clothes were clean and neat.
2. **Physical appearance**
   Client's appearance was age appropriate.
3. **General self-presentation**
   Client appeared nervous to engage in therapy and asked questions about how it should proceed and if he was doing well.
4. **Nature of typical relationship (dependent, submissive, aggressive, dominant, withdrawing, etc.)**
   Client described generally being more passive until someone "sets me off." It appears he engages in passive-aggressive behaviors to garner attention from those he loves when he is not receiving affection in a way or to the level that he desires.

5. **Behavior toward clinician (therapeutic alliance)**
   Client was polite and respectful toward clinician. Client appeared willing to work and once told clinician, "This is more relaxed than at the hospital."

Environmental Factors

1. **Elements in the environment, not already mentioned, that function as stressors to the client—those centrally related to the presenting problems and more peripheral.**
   None identified.
2. **Elements in the environment, not previously mentioned, that function as supports for clients (friends, family, recreational activities, etc.)**
   Client disclosed positive relationships at work.

Personality Dynamics

1. **Cognitive factors:**
   Client appears to employ logical fallacies when fighting with his spouse. He often withdraws into negative feedback loops until they reach a critical point and then he emotionally explodes. When his spouse does not respond in a caring and sympathetic way, he interprets this as confirmation of his negative thinking, and it further escalates his behaviors.
2. **Emotional factors:**
   Client has displayed a wide range of emotions within session and according to his own self-report. This becomes particularly problematic when he becomes stuck in a depressive state. He described becoming withdrawn.
3. **Behavior factors such as psychosomatic symptoms and existence of problematic habits or mannerisms:**
   Client disclosed being physically aggressive by throwing objects, punching holes in walls, and so on. While in a depressive state, his eating and sleep habits deteriorate, and it can lead to suicidal ideation.

Life Transition/Adaptation Skills

1. **Coping skills:** Uses humor to deal with stressful situations. Also resorts to physical actions when angered.
2. **Social resources:** Mother is his primary social support. Has a few friends at work.
3. **Psychological resources:** Client says he is a hard-worker who always starts what he finishes.

Formal Diagnosis

Diagnosis:
F33.2 major depressive disorder, recurrent, severe without psychotic features
Differential Diagnoses:
F34.1 dysthymic disorder
F43.21 adjustment disorder with depressed mood

Diagnostic Rationale

Discussion of symptoms/criteria showing how client meets the diagnostic criteria for the diagnoses given above:

Client meets five of the nine criteria for a major depressive episode, including depressed mood, diminished interest, hypersomnia, feelings of worthlessness, and recurrent thoughts of death. Because of the reoccurring nature of these episodes, it qualifies as major depressive disorder. With the inclusion of suicidality and recent hospitalization, the severity was assessed as severe. Client denied psychotic features.

- Include the differential diagnoses, demonstrating you ruled out at least two other diagnoses.

F34.1 Dysthymic Disorder

Though client discussed not being happy for a long time, his mood has been normal and jovial at times in session. He does not meet the sustained mild depressed state required for a diagnosis of dysthymic disorder.

F43.21 Adjustment Disorder with Depressed Mood

Because of the extended nature of his depressive episodes over the course of several years and the lack of a specific stressor to instigate the disorder.

Theoretical Conceptualization of the Case

The clinician is using a mindfulness-based cognitive behavioral therapy (MB-CBT) approach with the client. This approach utilizes techniques such as mindfulness, meditating, reflection, and grounding to address aspects of both the client's being and doing. In keeping with other CBT approaches, identification of cognitive distortions and logical fallacies is a primary concern for reframing. In addition, positive psychology aspects of supplementation of positive affirmations look at holistically addressing client wellness in addition to cessation of symptomology.

For this particular client, there are two presenting concerns. The first is regarding his self-described "funks," which meet the criteria of being major depressive episodes. MB-CBT was specifically designed to address the cyclical nature of depression. By being mindful of one's depressive triggers and coping behaviors, they are able to intervene and redirect the mood and behaviors in productive ways. For this particular client, identifying which moods and behaviors typically occur as a funk begins and what occurs during the episode will be particularly relevant. In addition, continued examination of his thinking patterns and how to reframe and redirect them will be important.

In approaching this particular client, the clinician is taking into consideration multiple aspects of culture. First, being a Black male immigrant presents particular experiences and challenges this clinician has not encountered in life. It will be important to mindfully reflect on any biases and work to empathetically understand the client's worldview. In addition, some Christian backgrounds can be resistant to MB-CBT techniques due to their connection to Far East religions and New Age philosophies. That said, Ethiopian

Tewahedo practices have included meditation and mindfulness practices as well. The client has shared he is open to the use of these techniques, particularly if they will help him to reach his goals. Finally, the clinician must actively engage with the client to ensure assumptions regarding cognitive distortions are accurate from the client's perspective as well.

Recommendations

- **Prognosis:** Currently, the client's prognosis is fair. He appears to be willing to make changes, but his history of mental health issues and their severity suggest it will be difficult to find a healthy balance.
- **Should services continue to be offered, or would a referral for counseling services elsewhere be more appropriate?**
  At this time, it is recommended that the client continue with weekly, individual sessions utilizing a MB-CBT approach. Referral to group counseling may be more appropriate once he has completed stabilization and is integrating interventions into daily practice.
- **Potential referral(s) to other professions (e.g., medical, psychiatric, etc.):**
  No referrals at this time.

CASE OF SUSAN (ENTIRE CASE IN CHAPTER 2)

CASE CONCEPTUALIZATION

Client Demographic Data

1. Susan Woods
2. Age 43, DOB 10/24/1980
3. Female
4. Single
5. 3 children, aged 9, 7, and 6. Children all live with client.
6. Client owns her home and lives in the home with her three children.

Socioeconomic Status Data

1. Full-time student
2. Client Income: 50,000/year
3. Education: Bachelor's degree in psychology, working on master's in counseling
4. Family members' education: Children are all in school and doing well; middle child has been diagnosed with ADHD.
5. Average family income: client's mother's income $80,000/year
6. Transportation status: owns own vehicle
7. Other economic resources: Client's mother lives in the area and is an emotional and social support to client. Client indicated that there was a time when the relationship was strained but that it is better now.
8. Economic stressors: Student loans and some personal/credit card debt. Student loans are currently paused, as client has returned to school, but client is worried about the payments resuming once she is done with school.

Presenting Problem(s): Include a description of the problem areas, listed separately, from the client's perspective, particularly noting client's view of their order of importance. Suggested items of focus:

1. **Were there precipitating factors?**
   Husband passed away suddenly 3 years ago due to an accidental drug overdose. Client indicated that she had no idea that he was abusing his prescription medication and that his overdose and death were very traumatic for her and the family.
2. **How long have the problems persisted?**
   3 years, since husband died from a drug overdose.
3. **Have problems previously occurred?**
   Client denied feeling this kind of anxiety and depression before husband's fatal drug overdose.
   What were the circumstances?
   N/A

4. **In what way, if any, do the problems relate to each other**?
   Client grieving husband and, in response, decided to become an addictions counselor in order to help people dealing with addiction and similar issues.
5. **Presence of suicide risk or ideation?**
   Client denies suicidal thoughts and/or ideations and states, "Our children need me more than ever" and "I know that my husband didn't want or mean to die and would want me to be strong, especially for the children."

Relevant History

1. **Family and relationship history**
   Client is a 43-year-old, heterosexual, White woman, with three children ages 9, 7, and 6. Client was married to husband for 8 years before he passed away from an accidental drug overdose 3 years ago. Client denies history of domestic abuse. Client is now enrolled in a CACREP-accredited master's degree program for addictions counseling, which she moved from another state to attend and be closer to family. Client has a good relationship with her mother, who helps with the children so that client can work and be in the counseling program. Client denies that she is dating, saying that "I don't have time to date, and if even if I did, I am not ready or interested."
2. **Cultural history and identity (issues of ethnicity and race, identification/acculturation)**
   Client denies any issues related to ethnicity of race, indicating that she is an "average White girl."
3. **Educational history (childhood/developmental, adulthood/current status)**
   Client met or exceeded all her developmental markers growing up. Client denies having any significant medical history and states that she was never hospitalized for anything growing up. Client graduated from high school on time and went on to earn a bachelor's degree in psychology at a large state university. Client met her husband after college and dated for several years before getting married in a small ceremony with friends and family.
4. **Vocational history (types, stability, satisfaction)**
   Client worked part time as a restaurant server during college and after college worked doing direct care in an adolescent treatment care facility with teenagers with behavioral and emotional issues.
5. **Medical history (acute/chronic illness, hospitalizations, surgeries, major patterns of illness in family, accidents, injuries, with whom/where/how often receive medical care, etc.)**
   Client denies hospitalizations of any kind, no family illness or personal trauma, client grew up with one older sibling who is 2 years older than her. Client denies abuse or issues with husband and states that he used marijuana when he was younger and was not using at the time when they met and got together. Client states that husband became addicted to pain pills after minor oral surgery.
6. **Health practices (sleeping, eating patterns, use of tobacco, consumption of caffeine, etc.)**
   Client has a history of sleep problems, including interrupted sleep and not being able to fall or stay asleep. Client has a history of disordered eating, sometimes binge eats.

7. **Mental health history (prior problems, symptoms, diagnoses, evaluations, therapy experiences, past prescribed medications, current and family-of-origin mental health histories)**
   Prior to husband's passing, client had no mental health issues or diagnoses. Client denies ever being on any prescribed medication for depression or anxiety. Client denies alcohol or marijuana use.
8. **Current medications (dosages, purposes, physician, compliance, effects, side effects, etc.)**
   Client indicates that she is not currently on any medication, sometimes takes a sleep aid.
9. **Legal history (arrests, DUI, jail/prison, lawsuits, any pending legal actions)**
   Client denies any arrests, DUIs, legal history.
10. **Use/misuse of alcohol or drugs (prescription or illegal)**
    Client denies use of alcohol or drugs.
11. **Family (current and origin) alcohol/drug history**
    Client indicated that her dad used to drink alcohol when she was growing up.

Interpersonal Factors

This section contains a description of client's orientation toward others in environment.

1. **Manner of dress**
   Client dressed in casual business clothes during initial session.
2. **Physical appearance**
   Client appeared to be a 43-year-old White female.
3. **General self-presentation**
   Client presented well, in business casual clothing, neat appearance.
4. **Nature of typical relationship (dependent, submissive, aggressive, dominant, withdrawing, etc.)**
   Client indicated that she has a natural submissive style in relationships but that she would like to work on being more assertive and independent.
5. **Behavior toward clinician (therapeutic alliance)**
   Client was polite and respectful toward clinician. Client indicated that she appreciates an open and direct style of communication.

Environmental Factors

1. **Elements in the environment, not already mentioned, that function as stressors to the client—those centrally related to the presenting problems and more peripheral.**
   Children were very young at the time of husband's passing, which added to client's stress, as client had been a stay-at-home mom at the time while husband worked full time to support the family. Client indicated that "my whole life was turned upside down and I had to care for my children, who had suddenly lost their father and figure out how I was going to support my family."
2. **Elements in the environment, not previously mentioned, that function as supports for clients (friends, family, recreational activities, etc.)**
   Client draws support from family, including mom.

Personality Dynamics

1. **Cognitive factors: data related to thinking and mental processes, such as intelligence, mental alertness, persistence of negative cognitions, positive cognitions, nature and content of fantasy life, level of insight (awareness of changes in feelings, behavior, reactions of others, understanding of the interplay, etc.), and capacity for judgment (ability to make decisions and carry out practical affairs of daily living)**

   Client acknowledged to falling into a pattern of negative thinking, where she catastrophizes and ruminates, exacerbating her anxiety and grief.

2. **Emotional factors, such as typical or most common emotional stress, predominant mood during interviews, appropriateness of affect, range of emotions client can display, cyclical aspects of client's emotional life.**

   Sadness: Client's deep sadness due to the loss of her husband seems to be a primary emotional response. This sadness might be pervasive and affect other areas of her life.

   Loneliness: Client may be feeling an acute sense of loneliness and isolation following her husband's death.

   Anger: Client may be experiencing anger toward her husband, herself, or the circumstances surrounding his death.

   Guilt: Client may feel guilty about things left unsaid or undone, or about how she is coping with her loss.

3. **Behavior factors, such as psychosomatic symptoms and existence of problematic habits or mannerisms.**

   Avoidance Behaviors

   Social Withdrawal: Client may be avoiding social interactions, isolating herself from friends, family, and peers.

   Academic Procrastination: Client might be delaying or avoiding her schoolwork, leading to increased stress and anxiety about her academic performance.

   Coping Mechanisms

   Maladaptive Coping: Client may be engaging in behaviors such as excessive sleeping, substance use, or binge-watching Netflix to escape her feelings.

   Adaptive Coping: Client may benefit from positive behaviors, such as seeking support from friends, attending therapy sessions, and engaging in hobbies or activities.

   Routine and Structure

   Disrupted Routine: The loss of client's husband and the stress of grad school may have disrupted client's daily routine, leading to irregular sleep patterns, eating habits, and exercise routines.

   Lack of Structure: Without a structured routine, client may struggle to manage her time effectively, contributing to feelings of being overwhelmed.

Health-Related Behaviors

Neglecting self-care: Client may be neglecting her physical health, such as skipping meals, not exercising, or failing to attend medical appointments.

Sleep Disturbances: Irregular sleep patterns, insomnia, or excessive sleeping can be behavioral manifestations of client's emotional state.

Emotional Expression

Suppressing Emotions: Client may be suppressing her emotions, avoiding expressing her grief and anxiety, which may exacerbate her distress.

Overreacting: Conversely, client may possibly be experiencing heightened emotional reactions, such as irritability or crying spells, in response to minor stressors, which could be leading to increased anxiety and distress.

Formal Diagnosis

Diagnosis:

F43.23 Adjustment disorder with mixed anxiety and depressed mood

Differential Diagnoses:

F41.1 Generalized anxiety disorder

F32 Major depressive disorder

Diagnostic Rationale

- **Discussion of symptoms/criteria showing how client meets the diagnostic criteria for the diagnoses given above.**

Adjustment disorder is characterized by the development of emotional or behavioral symptoms in response to an identifiable stressor (or stressors) occurring within 3 months of the onset of the stressor(s). The symptoms or behaviors are clinically significant as evidenced by one or more of the following:

1. Marked distress that is out of proportion to the severity or intensity of the stressor, considering the external context and cultural factors.
2. Significant impairment in social, occupational, or other important areas of functioning.

- Include the differential diagnoses, demonstrating you ruled out at least two other diagnoses.

F41.1 Generalized Anxiety Disorder: Client's anxiety is specifically linked to identifiable stressors rather than being chronic and generalized.

F32 Major Depressive Disorder: While client exhibits symptoms of depression, symptoms appear directly related to specific stressors rather than a pervasive mood disorder.

F43.81 Prolonged Grief Disorder: While normal grief could explain some of client's symptoms, her level of distress and impairment may exceed what is typically expected in normal bereavement, justifying a diagnosis of adjustment disorder.

Theoretical Conceptualization of the Case

Reality therapy is used in this case conceptualization.

Client is experiencing significant emotional distress following the death of her husband due to a drug overdose. She is having difficulties in her life transition and in coping with the demands of her graduate counseling program.

Background, including her relationship with her late husband and her current state of mind.

Assessment and Behavioral Observation:
It is important to observe and understand Susan's actions, choices, and their impact on her well-being.

Susan's description of her current challenges, feelings of loss, and difficulties in her academic program are critical for clinician to understand as counselor begins to establish a therapeutic relationship with Susan.

Basic Needs:

We can use reality therapy to conceptualize what may going on with Susan:

Susan's behavior is aimed at fulfilling five basic needs: love and belonging, power, freedom, fun, and survival. Understanding how her current situation affects these needs is crucial.

Current Behavior: Focus on what Susan is doing currently that is either helping or hindering her satisfaction of these needs.
Choice and Responsibility: Emphasize Susan's ability to make choices and take responsibility for her actions to improve her life situation.

Conduct Basic Needs Assessment:
Love and Belonging: Susan's sense of connection has been severely impacted by her husband's death. She may feel isolated and disconnected.
Power: Susan might feel powerless over her emotions and academic challenges.
Freedom: The sudden change in her life circumstances might make Susan feel trapped and restricted.
Fun: Grief and stress might have reduced Susan's engagement in enjoyable activities.
Survival: The stress and emotional turmoil could be affecting Susan's physical health and well-being.

Current Choices and Behaviors:
How is Susan currently attempting to cope with her loss? What behavior is she currently doing or engaged in? Are these behaviors helping her meet her basic needs effectively?

Perception:
Explore Susan's perception of her situation. Reality therapy posits that how we perceive our world influences our actions. Helping Susan to shift her perceptions can be key in her treatment through the lens of reality therapy.

Treatment Plan Using Reality Therapy
Goals
Short-term: Help Susan stabilize her emotional state and find immediate ways to cope with her grief and academic stress.
Long-term: Empower Susan to make effective choices that enhance her life satisfaction and fulfill her basic needs.

Interventions:
WDEP System:

Wants: Help Susan to clarify what she wants in her personal and academic life. What does she want to change?
Doing: Examine what Susan is currently doing to achieve her wants. Are her current behaviors effective?
Evaluation: Help Susan evaluate whether her current behaviors are getting her what she wants and meeting her basic needs.
Planning: Collaborate with Susan to create a specific, attainable plan (SAMIC3: Simple, Attainable, Measurable, Immediate, Controlled, Consistent, Committed) for changing her behaviors to meet her needs more effectively.

Emphasize building a supportive and trusting relationship between Susan and the clinician to provide a safe environment for her to explore her feelings and choices.
Focus on Present and Future: Rather than dwelling on past events, focus on what Susan can do now and moving forward to improve her situation.

Encourage Positive Actions: Encourage Susan to engage in activities that promote well-being and connection, such as joining support groups, reconnecting with friends, or finding new hobbies.

Here is an example WDEP application for this scenario:

Wants: Susan wants to feel more emotionally stable, succeed in her graduate program, and find a sense of normalcy after her husband's death.
Doing: Susan is currently isolating herself, struggling with her coursework, and experiencing intense grief.
Evaluation: Susan realizes that her current behaviors, while understandable, are not helping her achieve her goals or meet her basic needs effectively.
Planning: Susan and her clinician develop a plan that includes (1) setting aside time each day for self-care and relaxation, (2) joining a grief support group to connect with others who understand her loss, (3) developing a study schedule that balances her academic responsibilities with self-care, and (4) identifying and engaging in activities that bring her joy and fulfillment.

By focusing on these steps, reality therapy can help Susan to take practical, actionable steps to regain control over her life, meet her basic needs, and work toward a more fulfilling future.

Recommendations

- **Prognosis:**
  Positive prognostic indicators:
  Strong support system
  Access to family, friends, and support groups can significantly aid in recovery.
  Motivation for Therapy
  Client's engagement and willingness to engage in therapy are critical for positive outcomes.
  No History of Chronic Mental Health Issues
  Absence of long-standing mental health conditions can lead to quicker recovery.
- **Should services continue to be offered, or would a referral for counseling services elsewhere be more appropriate?**
  Client may benefit from continued counseling services and perhaps attending counseling biweekly or once per month to check in and review progress on coping skills and overall functioning.
- Potential referral(s) to other professions (e.g., medical, psychiatric, etc.):

No referrals at this time.

- Recommendation for a specific therapeutic orientation to be used with this client.
  Cognitive behavioral therapy or reality therapy
- Nature of treatment (e.g., specific clinician, priority of treatment issues, interaction with client characteristics such as defensiveness, motivation for treatment, problem complexity, etc.):
  N/A
- Format recommendations concerning working with the client (e.g., individual, group therapy, etc.):
  Client may benefit from both individual and group therapy at this time.

REFERENCES

Beck, J. (1995). *Cognitive therapy: Basics and beyond.* Guilford Press.

Cipani, E., & Golden, J. A. (2007). Differentiating behavioral & traditional case formulations for children with severe behavioral & emotional problems. *International Journal of Behavioral Consultation and Therapy, 3*(4), 537–545.

Cronin, T. J., Lawrence, K. A., Taylor, K., Norton, P. J., & Kazantzis, N. (2015). Integrating between-session interventions (homework) in therapy: The importance of the therapeutic relationship and cognitive case conceptualization. *Journal of Clinical Psychology: In Session, 71*(5), 439–450.

Easden, M. H., & Kazantzis, N. (2016). Case conceptualization research in cognitive behavior therapy: A state of the science review. *Journal of Clinical. Psychology, 74*, 356–384.

Falvey, J. E. (2001). Clinical judgment in case conceptualization and treatment planning across mental health disciplines. *Journal of Counseling & Development, 79*, 292–303.

Falvey, J. E., Bray, T. E., & Hebert, D. J. (2005). Case conceptualization and treatment planning: Investigation of problem-solving and clinical judgment. *Journal of Mental Health Counseling, 27*(4), 348–372.

Gazzillo, F., Dimaggio, G., & Curtis, J. T. (2021). Case formulation and treatment planning: How to take care of relationship and symptoms together. *Journal of Psychotherapy Integration, 31*(2), 115–128.

Groenier, M., Pieters, J. M., Witteman, C. L. M., & Lehmann, S. R. S. (2014). The effect of client case complexity on clinical decision making. *European Journal of Psychological Assessment, 30*(2), 150–158. https://doi.org/10.1027/1015-5759/a000184

Hagmayer, Y., Witteman, C., & Claes, L. (2021). PACT: A protocol for assessment, mechanism-based case formulation and treatment planning. *Journal of Evaluation in Clinical Practice, 27*, 648–656.

Healthcare Providers Service Organization. (2019, March). *Counselor liability claim report (2nd ed.).* https://www.hpso.com/getmedia/ac13a1d8-3bdd-4117-ad36-8fba7c419153/counselor-claim-report-second-edition.pdf

Hurst, J. C., & McKinley, D. L. (1988). An ecological diagnostic classification plan. Journal of Counseling and Development, 66(5), 228-232.

Lake, A. J., Rodriguez-Quintana, N., Lewis, C. C., & Brothers, B. M. (2022). ADDRESSING diversity: Clinical assessment and outcomes in a psychology training clinic. *Training and Education in Professional Psychology, 16*(1), 229–234.

Lehman, B. J., David, D. M., & Gruber, J. A. (2017). Rethinking the biopsychosocial model of health: Understanding health as a dynamic system. *Social & Personality Psychology Compass, 11*(8), 1–17. https://doi.org/10.1111/spc3.12328.

Lenz, A. S., & Litam, S. D. A. (2023). Integrating the social determinants of mental health Into case conceptualization and treatment planning. *Journal of Counseling Development, 101*, 416–428.

Macneil, C. A., Hasty, M. K., Conus, P., & Berk, M. (2012). Is diagnosis enough to guide interventions in mental health? Using case formulation in clinical practice. *BMC Medicine, 10*(111), 1–3.

Maniacci, M. P., Carlson, J., & Sackett-Maniacci, L. (2017). Neo-Adlerian approaches to psychotherapy. *Journal of Individual Psychology, 73*(2), 95–109.

Neufeldt, S. A., Pinterits, E. J., Moleiro, C. M., Lee, T. E., Yang, P. H., & Brodie, R. E. (2006). How do graduate student therapists incorporate diversity factors in case conceptualization? *Psychotherapy: Theory, Research, Practice, Training, 43*(4), 464–479

Osborn, C. J., Dean, E. P., & Petruzzi, M. L. (2004). Use of simulated multidisciplinary treatment teams and client actors to teach case conceptualization and treatment planning skills. *Counselor Education & Supervision, 44*, 121–134.

Prieto, L. R., & Scheel, K. R. (2002). Using case documentation to strengthen counselor trainees' case conceptualization skills. *Journal of Counseling & Development, 80*, 11–21.

Sperry, L. (2005a). Case conceptualization: A strategy for incorporating individual, couple, and family dynamics in the treatment process. *The American Journal of Family Therapy, 33*, 189–194.

Sperry, L. (2005b). Case conceptualization: The missing link between theory and practice. *The Family Journal: Counseling and Therapy for Couples and Families, 13*(1), 71–76.

Sperry, L. (2017). Similarities between cognitive behavior therapy and Adlerian psychotherapy: Assessment, case conceptualization, and treatment. *The Journal of Individual Psychology, 73*(2), 110–123.

Sperry, L., & Sperry, J. (2020). *Case conceptualization: Mastering this competency with ease and confidence* (2nd ed.). Routledge.

CHAPTER 7

Treatment Planning

Melinda Mays, EdD, Holly J. Mattingly, PhD, Mona Gallo, EdD, Gregory L. Bohner, PhD, and Daniel R. Romero, PhD

INTRODUCTION

The treatment plan is typically the most used document from the client's file. Even though there is little guidance from the research to guide clinicians on treatment plans, it is critical that attention be paid to every detail (Gutierrez et al., 2018; Wiger, 2012). Treatment planning is an integral part of a client's service. The treatment record is a vital collection of data regarding the clinician's assessment of their client's needs and concerns and the treatment provided. The treatment plan should be based on the client's reported symptoms and subsequent diagnosis after a thorough intake assessment. When developing a treatment plan, clinicians are ethically obligated to use evidence-based techniques and procedures that are firmly grounded in scientific theory (American Counseling Association [ACA], 2014).

Some clinicians see the creation of a treatment plan as an arduous process whose only purpose is to satisfy the demands of third-party payers, often referred to as *managed care*. Over the course of time, managed care has become the gatekeeper of mental health practice (Falvey et al., 2005). But whether a clinician is meeting the requirements of managed care or providing services to a client without insurance reimbursement, a properly executed treatment plan can be of great benefit for both the client and the clinician.

Managed care, most licensing bodies, as well as mental health associations (ACA, American Psychological Association [APA], National Association of Social Work [NASW]) clarify that the client needs to know what is involved in their decision to engage in the counseling process. While the informed consent would address many legal and ethical concerns, the treatment plan is needed to provide information as to the likely duration of counseling and the expected rate of client improvement so they can make an informed decision with consideration of their financial and personal resources. This allows the level of commitment of the client to be factored into the decision-making (Hatchett, 2020).

There is a wide variety of formats for developing a treatment plan. Most agencies adopt a generic treatment plan format that will meet the needs of their clients, as well as third-party payers. It is beyond the scope of this text to address all the variations that one might encounter. However, the components are usually very consistent, including problem statements, goal statements, objectives and interventions, and a timeline for those (Wubbolding et al., 2017).

ETHICAL CONSIDERATIONS OF TREATMENT PLANNING

Part of a clinician's professional responsibility is to ensure that proper ethical procedures are followed at every step of treatment. This includes treatment planning. Although not every code of ethics specifically mentions treatment planning, the implications are clear. Whether explicitly stated or implied, a well-formulated and well-documented treatment plan is an essential ethical duty of the mental health clinician.

Clinicians need to develop timely and adequate documentation to provide uninterrupted services (ACA, 2014). Since the purpose of the treatment plan is to define the delivery and continuity of services, it is obvious that the written treatment plan and its components are an ethical duty. The *2014 ACA Code of Ethics* (ACA, 2014) stresses the necessity of collaboration between client and clinician and the importance of considering the abilities, temperament, developmental level and circumstances of the client.

The *APA Ethical Principles of Psychologists and Code of Conduct* (APA, 2017) states that clinicians are to create, manage, keep, distribute, and destroy records and data in conjunction with their professional work. These guidelines are in place to assist a clinician in facilitating the means for client services by the original clinician or by other professionals. In addition, clinicians guided by the APA use their records to meet institutional requirements, establish accuracy for billing and payments, and ensure compliance with the law.

Although the *Code of Ethics of the National Association of Social Workers* (NASW, 2021) does not explicitly address treatment planning, it is stressed that the primary responsibility of clinicians is to promote the well-being of clients. In general, clients' interests are central. In addition, the clinician is to respect and promote the right of clients to self-determination and assist clients in their efforts to identify and clarify their goals.

The most specific language regarding treatment planning comes from the *Code of Ethics for the National Board for Certified Counselors* (National Board for Certified

Counselors, 2023). The guidance is that the clinician will work in conjunction with the client to develop a written treatment plan that includes attainable goals with appropriate techniques that meet the client's psychological and physical capacity and needs. In addition, clinicians are guided to update and modify the treatment plan when changes occur in the client's treatment. The changes that could occur may be related to goals, roles, techniques, and diagnoses. Lastly, if such changes do in fact need to occur, clinicians are required to obtain the client's written approval for such changes.

LEGAL CONSIDERATIONS OF TREATMENT PLANNING

Good documentation contained in the counseling record is necessary for both the client's welfare and the protection of the counselor (Piazza & Baruth, 1990). Overall, licensure laws are specifically focused on protecting the client. A well-developed treatment plan is an excellent way of ensuring the client's treatment needs and goals are the primary focus for the clinician and that the client is being safeguarded in their treatment process. The development of a comprehensive treatment plan requires the active involvement of the client and would include the client's strengths, needs, resilience, functioning, and readiness for change, as well as a substantiated diagnosis and inclusion of both short-term and long-range goals specific to the client (Kelly, 2023).

It is imperative for the clinician to adhere to a set of guidelines that also meets the ethical and legal requirements for the benefit of clients. There are federal government regulations related to treatment planning. Specifically, the Centers for Medicare and Medicaid Services emphasize that treatment plans must be individualized, based on the client's strengths and disabilities, have a substantiated diagnosis, and include short-term and long-range goals (Kelly, 2023). Generally, clinicians working in community mental health centers (CMHCs) are required to have a person-centered active treatment plan that evolves from a comprehensive individualized assessment. The treatment plan should demonstrate the care and treatment services that will be utilized to address the client's biopsychosocial, physical, emotional, and therapeutic needs and goals (Cornell Law School, 2023).

Each state may also have specific regulations related to treatment planning. For the states that do, most follow the regulations required for CMHCs. The regulations for CMHCs include utilizing the results of any assessments and regularly reviewing the treatment plan with the client and documentation of any changes needed to the treatment plan (check your state's laws because some states require a specific timeframe for review). The CMHC regulations also require a clinician to document the client's progress or lack thereof, as well as the discussions with clients and their stakeholders (as applicable) about the client's treatment experience. In addition, clinicians are required to document the techniques and methods that will be utilized to assist the client in reducing and/or eliminating symptoms and to identify measurable objectives and goals, along with the type, duration, and frequency of services recommended to assist the client in reaching said goals. In addition, the CMHC regulations also require the treatment plan be signed and dated by the client, as well as any applicable stakeholders. Whether the clinician's state's laws require the treatment plan to be signed and dated by the client or not, we strongly recommend that the clinician retrieve the client's dated signature on the treatment plan as evidence of the client's informed consent and buy in to treatment. Lastly, the CMHC regulations note that a copy of the treatment plan be provided to the client, with some states making this a requirement.

INSURANCE PURPOSES IN DEVELOPING AND DOCUMENTING A TREATMENT PLAN

As previously mentioned, third-party payers usually have their own rules and regulations as to the development, formatting, and maintenance of treatment plans (Wiger, 2012; Wubbolding et al., 2017). One of the significant requirements of most third-party payers is related to the use of specific language. Since these entities have a primary concern of ensuring that services provided are appropriate and efficient, the language of the treatment plan must be specific. The terms "observable" and "measurable" are usually used to define the type of language that should be used for objectives. Vague terms such as "increase," "improve," and the like could mean anything from an insignificant gain to a major improvement. A main concern of using unclear or vague language in the treatment plan is that the objective may be met without meeting the intent (Wiger, 2012).

Another important point of language use is in describing the desired behavior. Using nonspecific or nonmeasurable language, such as "improving social skills" or "increasing self-esteem," in objectives is not advised, as it has constructs that are not easily quantified (Wiger, 2012). It is much more appropriate to designate observable behaviors that would be indicative of those constructs (Piazza & Baruth, 1990). For example, "improving social skills" could be revised to include a specific number of social interactions, such as "Will improve social skills through six separate social interactions."

Unfortunately, third-party payers often have a strong influence on how many sessions a client can attend. Many clients are unable to privately pay for counseling services, which may limit clinicians. Clinicians must consider the client's financial limitations when planning for termination. If a client is limited to a specified number of counseling sessions, then it is in the client's best interest to design the treatment plan with the realistic expectation of what the client might accomplish given those limits.

THE PURPOSES OF DEVELOPING A TREATMENT PLAN

Although there is very little in the literature regarding exactly what information should be included in the treatment plan, there are some clear purposes for it. The primary purpose of generating a well-developed treatment plan is for the benefit of the client (Seligman, 1993). But for the clinician, the treatment plan helps develop accountability by monitoring and determining the best course of action (Wiger, 2012). Optimally, the treatment plan is a way to track a client's progress and can be used to identify the purpose, provide structure, and define anticipated results to the counseling process (Gutierrez et al., 2018; Piazza & Baruth, 1990; Seligman, 1993). Other purposes for the development of a treatment plan include meeting legal obligations, providing a layer of protection for the clinician, as well as acting as a potential avenue to communicate with other professionals regarding the client care (Gopi et al., 2019).

Over time, there has been a strong push for limiting treatment to what is considered evidence-based treatment. One school of thought is to develop the treatment plan using the diagnosis as the focus and applying a prescribed plan of action. While research has yielded some very helpful direction in becoming more efficient in choosing appropriate treatments, there is some discussion about over reliance on these findings in lieu of other factors that should also be included in the clinician's clinical reasoning. It is suggested that decisions regarding the client's treatment are constructed utilizing a wide variety of inputs, including not only research findings but also factors such as clinician observations and assessments and the experiential knowledge of the clinician (Shapiro, 2009). In all, it is more beneficial to the client to base the treatment plan on a well-developed case conceptualization (see Chapter 6) of the client's unique situation (Gazzillo et al., 2021, Falvey et al., 2005, Restifo, 2011).

There is an emerging interest in stressing prevention through early interventions and alternative methods of remediation rather than mainly focusing on the diagnosis. Included in this is the use of the "wheel of wellness," which addresses a life balance in several areas of life. Although there are several variations of this model, important areas to consider in developing the treatment plan include spirituality, self-direction, work and leisure, friendship, and love (Myers et al., 2000).

THE IMPORTANCE OF DOCUMENTATION

A detailed treatment plan is one of the most consulted pieces of documentation in a client record. It outlines not only the indicated problems and desired outcomes (goals) but also the steps to achieve these (objectives) and the clinician's role in the process (interventions). The specific language of the plan defines the measurements that allow both the client and the clinician to monitor progress during treatment. The use of clinical judgment is critical and can be documented by including supporting details. The treatment plan should be written in objective language that is easily understood by the client, avoiding demeaning terminology and jargon that can cause harm and create confusion (Gopi et al., 2019). The treatment plan should not be altered once it is created and signed. The treatment plan can be amended or a whole new treatment plan designed, if there is clear documentation of the reason for the change.

JUSTIFICATION OF TREATMENT

Agencies, third-party payers, and some licensing laws require the clinician to justify the client's treatment. The treatment plan is a distinct way to provide evidence and justification for the client's treatment. Clinicians are encouraged to consider several basic areas that are best to include on the client's treatment plan.

Defining the Problem or Area of Change

Most health treatment, even mental health treatment, has historically operated in the paternalism model—sometimes referred to as the *doctor-knows-best model*, in which the clinician makes the critical decisions with little client input. It is becoming more common to use a collaborative model, providing more opportunities for client input. This has been shown to produce better client adherence to treatment, increased satisfaction, greater symptom reduction, lower rates of therapy, and a perception of a higher level of care (Pham et al., 2019).

Some clients come to counseling with a clear understanding of themselves, their situation, and what they want from the counseling process. Others come in with little self-awareness and only a vague sense of the direction they wish to pursue. Most clients fall somewhere between these two extremes. It is the job of the clinician to work collaboratively with the client to clarify the wants and needs of the clients and clearly define those into problem statements. Although it is best to document the defined problems on a treatment plan, some treatment plan formats do not require the problem statements to be written on the actual document. Either way, the conversations that clearly define the identified problems are very important, as they form the basis of the treatment plan (Piazza & Baruth, 1990, Wiger, 2012).

SMART Goals and Objectives

Once the client's current situation has been assessed, the next step is to develop goal statements. Goal statements are critical for focus of the treatment plan (Wiger, 2012). It is similar to planning a trip. All the decisions that go into planning a trip are based on the destination. Things like what to pack, what type of transportation is needed, budget, and so on cannot be determined until the destination is clear. In the same way, the goal statements establish the destination of the treatment and then appropriate objectives and interventions can be determined. In fact, Seligman (1993) has compared the process of treatment planning to developing a road map.

New clinicians sometimes confuse the destination and the journey. They develop goal statements that are really objectives. A statement such as "Client will attend X number of therapy sessions" is not in itself a goal. A client can attend numerous sessions without experiencing any discernible change. The reason a clinician would state a client should attend sessions is because participating in those will hopefully bring about insights that lead to a behavioral change. That change would be the goal.

Mentioned prior, clinician and client collaboration is important in determining the problems to address. It is even more critical in the establishment of goals (Wiger, 2012). The client may enter treatment with well-thought-out goals. If so, then it is important that the clinician assesses their developmental and cultural appropriateness. If not, then the clinician may need to infer goals from the information provided by the client (Gazzillo et al., 2021).

It is important that the goals in the official treatment plan be clear to both the client and clinician. A helpful way to ensure this is the use of SMART goals. This is an acronym for the descriptors: specific, measurable, attainable/achievable, relevant/realistic and time-bound (Lee, 2010). This format for developing goals is becoming popular in a variety of areas, including mental health.

Using language that is specific is very important in writing goals. A well-developed treatment plan will include language that gives clear, measurable criteria for the goals and objectives. It is not helpful for the client and the clinician to have differing opinions on what is expected from treatment. While writing detailed goals may seem like unnecessary effort, the details are more likely to aid in client success. The clinician and client need clear direction (Lee, 2010).

The idea of a treatment planning goal being measurable may seem a bit too detailed for some clinicians. However, including criteria to measure the success, or lack thereof, adds to the clarity of the goal. It is much easier for a client to ascertain if a goal has been met when the criteria is clear. Goal attainment can be very motivating and develop momentum for tackling other goals.

One of the major roles of the clinician is to work with the client to develop goals that are achievable. Many clients come to counseling with only a vague idea of what they hope to accomplish. It is also important to consider the amount of time and resources a client can or would be willing to invest in the therapeutic process. In an ideal world, all clients would stay the needed number of sessions to reach their optimal success. Due to various reasons, some clients may not complete treatment. The client's circumstances and developmental concerns must be considered when deciding what the client can achieve in treatment (Gazzillo et al., 2021).

Another important factor to consider is how the client's goals are relevant to the client and their circumstances. The clinician needs to take care to help the client determine their own wishes and direction, apart from those of others. It will be difficult for a client to be committed to a goal that is not relative (Lee, 2010).

The final criteria is that the goal be time-bound (Lee, 2010). Not only is time-limited treatment required by many third-party payers but it also helps to add accountability to the treatment process. In addition, a clearly defined time frame may help the client see that counseling will not go on indefinitely and that there is a definite benefit on the horizon.

Objectives

Once goal statements have been established, the clinician and client will develop objectives. *Objectives* are incremental steps that lead to accomplishing the already established goals (Wiger, 2012). To continue with the previously mentioned trip analogy, once you know your destination, then it may become abundantly clear what to pack, how to get there, items to budget for, and so on. In the same way, once clear goal statements have been delineated, breaking those goals down into logical steps should become a straightforward process.

Objectives should be small enough to be attainable but also enough of a challenge to help the client feel that progress is being made. There is a "sweet spot" between objectives being too simple, which could lead the client to develop a lack of motivation, and objectives being too challenging, which could cause anxiety and avoidance (Piazza & Baruth, 1990; Wiger, 2012).

When writing appropriate objectives, it is important to consider more than just the desired behavior change. Many things can influence the client's ability to complete goals and develop a reasonable timeline. This includes things such as the client's motivations, insight, cooperation, and many more (Wiger, 2012). Objectives also need to be unambiguously worded, explicitly written, and clearly understood by the client. According to the language of the objective, it should be very clear whether the client has met the objective or not. Statements such as "The client will improve" would be hard to assess. This could reward only a token effort, or the client and clinician may disagree on whether enough improvement has been made to justify considering the objective accomplished. Since objectives are used to document client progress, both the client and clinician must have a clear understanding of how to determine when the objectives are met.

Interventions

Once the problems have been defined, goals developed, and objectives chosen, writing the interventions should be relatively easy. It is critical that the treatment plan clarifies and addresses the needs of the client. Formulating good goal statements and objectives should guarantee that the treatment plan does just that. The next step is for the clinician to add interventions to the treatment plan. *Interventions* are the specific strategies that the clinician will employ to assist the client in accomplishing the objectives and reaching the overall goals of the treatment plan. The chosen interventions are usually influenced by the theoretical orientation of the clinician (explored later in the chapter).

Timelines

Determining a timeline can be complicated. Setting an unrealistic timeline may discourage the client and lead to premature termination of services (Desrosiers et al., 2015). Therefore, it is imperative a clinician consider all the factors that can affect how long it takes a client to reach objectives and ultimately their goals. Internal factors such as motivation, the client's abilities or challenges, and the like will have an impact on the timeline. External factors such as personal responsibilities, financial obligations, third-party reimbursement, and so on can also impact the timeline of treatment. Because of the internal and external constraints, it is important that the treatment plan be a malleable document. The treatment plan should be subject to constant monitoring with opportunities to reevaluate and/or review the effectiveness of the plan (Piazza & Baruth, 1990).

One complication of developing a timeline for treatment comes from the involvement of third-party payers, particularly the requirement that the number of sessions be determined before or at the beginning of treatment. This may negatively impact the process of treatment in that the actual number of sessions needed may be more or less than the original estimate. This may cause clients to forego personal exploration to be sure that they have the time to address their most pressing issues, or the client may have resolved their problems sooner than expected and then the counseling may enter into a sort of limbo where it seems like the client is continuing to attend counseling to "get their money's worth" (Hoffman & Meier, 2001). It is important, then, that the clinician makes use of every opportunity to modify the number of sessions as needed and as allowed by the contract.

Since there is little research to guide the clinician's development of a timeline for treatment, the clinician must rely on their own knowledge and experience. This may not yield the most reliable basis of judgment because there is the tendency to remember those clients that stay longer more often than those that were of shorter duration or terminated treatment early. When determining timelines, clinicians often overestimate the typical duration of counseling. Generally, clients exhibit much more progress in the earlier sessions. In addition, acute problems will generally need fewer sessions than those with more chronic interpersonal and personality domain issues (Hatchett, 2020).

Termination

The last component of the treatment plan contains the criteria for discharge. This may be included as part of the goal or objective statements or listed as a separate item, depending on the treatment plan format. It is important for the clinician to begin counseling with the end of the client's treatment in mind (Covey, 2020). The criteria for discharge, often called *termination*, will quite often be stated in the original goal statements (Wiger, 2012).

Termination of counseling services should not only be the end but also a beginning. The client will be starting a new phase of life without the direct support of the clinician. In planning for termination, there also should be consideration for what the client will need beyond counseling. In this phase, the client should be prepared for what is to come and how they will manage on their own. The client should also be made aware of what resources will be available should the client find the need for them (see Chapter 9).

THE ROLE OF THEORY IN TREATMENT PLANNING

One of the things that separates clinicians from laypersons is the knowledge and application of theory. Clinicians have a wide range of possible theoretical orientations from which to choose. Although it is beyond the scope of this chapter to discuss all the possible theories that might guide treatment, there is some common ground for treatment addressed by all. These areas are assessment, treatment, and discharge. The assessment phase has the same focus for all clients, regardless of theory. The purpose is to determine the depth of the problem and whether the client would benefit from mental health services. It is usually at this stage that a diagnosis is formed (Wiger, 2012). The treatment phase is where the clinician's use of theory has an impact. The goals, objectives, and interventions of treatment will often follow the focus of the chosen theory. Some examples of how theory might appear in a treatment plan could be clarifying cognitions, increasing client insight, modifying behaviors, or focus on the future (Wiger, 2012). Regardless of the method, the ultimate goal is the client's success.

Counseling is both an art and a science. Most clinicians can be placed on a continuum that varies from viewing therapy as mostly or completely science-based to viewing therapy as mostly or completely an art. Many therapists define themselves as "eclectic," basing their choice on what is best for their client. Although not all therapies are the same, they all address common variables, including the theoretical relationship, cognitive insight and change, emotions in therapy, and client expectations (Wiger, 2012). The treatment plan can be constructed to address these important points, regardless of the theory preferred by the clinician for the client.

The clinician will use their knowledge of theory in conceptualizing the client's problems, patterns, and themes. Undoubtedly, this same process is reflected in some of the choices for objectives and interventions. However, the main purpose of the treatment plan is to ensure, sometimes to third-party payers, that the client and clinician maintain a continuity of care. This is also crucial if the client must be transferred to another clinician (Wiger, 2012). No matter the theory employed, care must be taken to construct the treatment plan in such a way that the aforementioned purposes will be met.

THE ROLE OF DIAGNOSIS IN TREATMENT PLANNING

The medical model of treatment is based on using the diagnosis to determine the course of treatment. The diagnosis is usually determined before treatment planning begins. Although there is much controversy about the role of diagnosis, it can be used by clinicians to guide treatment. It also is used by third-party payers to verify the need for medical care. The importance of diagnosis and the benefits of its inclusion in treatment planning should not be ignored.

There is ample research that addresses the effectiveness of a certain theory with a certain diagnosis. This research has mainly been driven by the desire to have evidence-based practice that guides mental health treatment. Along with the demand for evidence-based practices, the National Alliance on Mental Illness (n.d.) reports that many clients have feelings of relief and hope after receiving a diagnosis. Even though clients find simple relief in receiving a diagnosis, remember that simple diagnostic matching does not take into consideration many variables, such as context, client motivation, and process dynamics (Falvey et al., 2005). The diagnosis will not likely address response to previous treatment or limitations stemming from the realities of the client's life situation. This is where the clinician's expertise can address the many other factors that would influence the course and outcome, outside of diagnostic symptomatology, in treatment (Restifo, 2011).

THE IMPORTANCE OF CLIENT ENGAGEMENT

If the clinician strictly relied on a diagnosis to inform the treatment plan, it would potentially minimize the importance of including the client in the process. Listening to the client and any stakeholders ensures that what is important to the client and those in their world is built into the treatment plan. The doctor-knows-best model, popular prior to the 1980s, often left the client with feelings of lack of control and low involvement in decision-making and has been identified as a risk factor for having a negative experience in psychotherapy (Pham et al., 2019).

Engaging the client and any stakeholders in the treatment planning process is part of establishing therapeutic rapport and facilitating client empowerment (Wubbolding et al., 2017). It is imperative that clinicians consider family, friend, social, and community involvement in treatment planning as part of determining any causative factors, as well as a holistic approach to resolving some of the client's problems (Bertolote, 2008).

Since the client is the expert on their own values, emotions, barriers, and so on, including them in the treatment process may make them feel respected from the start of treatment. These notions are supported by numerous studies that show there are better outcomes related to greater client involvement in treatment, as well as better adherence to treatment and lower dropout rates (Pham et al., 2019).

REVISING A TREATMENT PLAN

Sometimes revisions need to be made in the treatment plan, especially when a significant change has occurred (Wiger, 2012). As the counseling relationship progresses, sometimes new issues surface. This may happen because the client needs to develop a higher level of trust before revealing them, or perhaps the client was unaware of their underlying pattern until engaging in self-exploration through counseling. Ongoing monitoring will ensure that, in such circumstances, the treatment plan will be revised to accommodate those changes. This can include merely revising objectives or goals, or possibly replacing objectives or goals that are no longer assisting the client in reaching their overall goal. It is important, as clients progress through the objectives, that both the client and clinician consider the need for revisions as necessary. These treatment plan updates are often required by third-party providers to demonstrate the effectiveness of the interventions (Wiger, 2012).

Another way of keeping the treatment plan current is through updates. These can be written in document form as a summary of objectives that have been met and those that are still in progress. Clinical notes are also a way to document that a treatment plan is being followed. Since the counseling sessions should be based on the treatment plan, it follows that documenting the session would also be documenting the progress, or lack thereof, the client has made on the treatment plan (Wiger, 2012).

CONCLUSION

Treatment planning needs to be an ongoing process that provides clarity to the counseling process. It is also an accountability measure for both the client and the clinician. The goal statements show that both the client and the clinician understand the focus of treatment. The objectives should clarify the expectations the client must meet to progress and reach those goals. The interventions are how the clinician will offer their expertise in the process. The timeline ensures that assessment of progress will occur and there are clear criteria to determine when termination is appropriate.

CASE OF ABEL (ENTIRE CASE IN CHAPTER 2)

Session #3

Abel comes to see you for his third session. He has rescheduled the past 2 weeks because of sickness. As Abel walks into the session, his eyes are downcast, and his nose is red. He apologizes for missing the past 2 weeks and thanks you for meeting with him. He shares that in the past couple of weeks, the fighting between him and his wife has intensified. The other night, Simon mentioned going to dinner with Mary and her friend from work Marcus. Simon also said Mary was laughing and smiling throughout the meal and was "happier than she has been in a long time." Abel says he is not sure what he wants to do moving forward, but he cannot stop thinking that Mary is cheating on him and maybe he should just get a divorce. When you explore the topic further, Abel denies that he has had any suicidal ideation, but he does think this has led to him being in a funk again. When you ask about his behavior the past few weeks, Abel shares that he has been drinking more and eating poorly. However, he insists that he was diagnosed with the flu a week and a half ago and that is why he has canceled appointments. Abel reiterates that he thinks the sessions with you are important and that he is committed to doing better. As you finish the session, Abel decides that one of his goals is to eat more healthy meals for lunch. Instead of stopping at a fast-food restaurant every day, he decides to make his lunch for 3 out of the 5 days. He also decides to spend at least one night with just him and Simon because his son "is the most important thing in the world."

TREATMENT PLAN

Client Name: Abel Tesfaye **Date:** 4/23/2024

PRESENTING PROBLEMS: Client is returning home after hospitalization from suicidal ideation and wants to address his depressive symptoms. In addition, he wants to improve the relationship with his spouse so that it becomes "more bearable."

***ICD-10* # DIAGNOSIS & SPECIFIER(s):** F33.2 major depressive disorder, recurrent, severe without psychotic features

***ICD-10* # DIFFERENTIAL DIAGNOSIS(es):** F34.1 dysthymic disorder

F43.21 adjustment disorder with depressed mood

TREATMENT PROCEDURES

1. Mode of therapy: Individual
2. Sessions per week expected: 1
3. Total number of sessions expected (including past sessions): 10–12

Problem 1: Client is experiencing depressive symptoms.

Goal 1: Learn three coping strategies to decrease depressive symptoms by 50% occurrences a week.

Date	Objectives	Projected Achievement Date	Clinical Intervention
4/23/2024	Increase client sense of balance when experiencing depressive symptoms.	5/21/2024	Teach client breathing techniques and monitor client perception of effectiveness for a month.
4/23/2024	Increase client sense of control when experiencing depressive symptoms.	5/21/2024	Teach client grounding techniques and monitor client perception of effectiveness for a month.
4/23/2024	Track symptomology for better client understanding of precipitating events.	5/21/2024	Review client journal in session to monitor mood and identify specific triggers for maladaptive behaviors.

Problem 2: Miscommunication with spouse is causing distress.

Goal 2: Increase positive communication patterns with spouse to three positive conversations a week.

Date	Objectives	Projected Achievement Date	Clinical Intervention
4/23/2024	Deescalate explosive conversations with spouse.	6/11/2024	Teach client use of "I-statements" and track usage over the course of a month.
4/23/2024	Improve client awareness of how he contributes to problem and how to alter his contributions.	6/18/2024	Identify patterns of cognitive distortions in session and reframe statements to productive sentiments.
4/23/2024	Provide positive experiences in addition to reducing negative experiences.	6/18/2024	Plan three date nights over the course of 2 months to increase positive engagement with spouse.

Clinician Signature: Tara Pist, MEd Date: 4/2/2024

Client Signature: Abel Tesfaye Date: 4/2/2024

CASE OF SUSAN (ENTIRE CASE IN CHAPTER 2)

TREATMENT PLAN

Client Name: Susan Woods **Date:** 6/10/2024

PRESENTING PROBLEMS: Client is experiencing anxiety and stress related to recent changes and life stressors. She has recently experienced the loss of spouse, significant move, new home, returned to being a full-time student after not expecting to ever return to school, change in income, change in life direction.

***ICD-10* # DIAGNOSIS & SPECIFIER(s):** F43.23 adjustment disorder with mixed anxiety and depressed mood

***ICD-10* # DIFFERENTIAL DIAGNOSIS(es):** F41.1 generalized anxiety disorder, F32 major depressive disorder

TREATMENT PROCEDURES

1. Mode of therapy: Individual
2. Sessions per week expected: 1
3. Total number of sessions expected (including past sessions): 10–12

Problem 1: Client is experiencing increase in anxiety.
Goal 1: Reduce anxiety to manageable levels.

Date	Objectives	Projected Achievement Date	Clinical Intervention
6/14/2024	Enhance understanding and acceptance of the loss.	7/5/2024	Initial assessment and relationship building/establish a trusting therapeutic relationship.
6/14/2024	Develop coping strategies to manage anxiety and grief.	7/5/2024	Collaborate with client, using empathic listening, open-ended questions, and validation of feelings.
6/14/2024	Improve daily functioning and emotional well-being.	7/5/2024	Use WDEP system (wants, doing, evaluation, planning). Wants: Explore goals, desires, and what client wishes to achieve. Doing: Help client to identify current actions and behaviors. Evaluation: Assess how these behaviors are helping or hindering progress. Planning: Collaborate with client to develop a practical plan for change.

Problem 2: Client is having problems focusing in her counseling program.
Goal 2: Stabilize and reduce academic stress.

Date	Objectives	Projected Achievement Date	Clinical Intervention
6/14/2024	Develop effective study and time management skills.	8/2/2024	Help client to develop a structured study schedule, including use of planners/calendars.
6/14/2024	Improve academic performance and confidence.	8/2/2024	Complete a comprehensive assessment of academic history, including study habits and stressors.
6/14/2024	Achieve a balanced and sustainable academic routine.	8/2/2024	Discuss the importance of self-care and balanced routines.

Problem 3: Client is grieving her relationship/partner/marriage.
Goal 3: Process and accept loss of husband.

Date	Objectives	Projected Achievement Date	Clinical Intervention
6/14/2024	Increase emotional supports and stabilize acute grief symptoms.	8/23/2024	Help client to understand grief process and normalize feelings and experiences.
6/14/2024	Explore and discover healthy expression and processing of grief.	8/23/2024	Provide information on the stages of grief.
6/14/2024	Achieve a sense of acceptance and integration of the loss.	8/23/2024	Provide a safe space for client to express feelings and feel validated and understood.

Clinician Signature: Gene Hudlow, MEd, LPCC   Date 6/14/2024

Client Signature: Susan Woods   Date: 6/14/2024

REFERENCES

American Counseling Association. (2014). *2014 ACA code of ethics.* https://www.counseling.org/docs/

American Psychological Association. (2017). *Ethical principles of psychologists and code of conduct.* https://www.apa.org/ethics/code

Bertolote, J. M. (2008). Mental health policy paper: The roots of the concept of mental health. *World Psychiatry, 7,* 113–116.

Cornell Law School. (2023, November 22). *42 CFR § 485.916 - Condition of participation: Treatment team, person-centered active treatment plan, and coordination of services.* Legal Information Institute. https://www.law.cornell.edu/cfr/text/42/485.916

Covey, S. R. (2020). *The 7 Habits of Highly Effective People.* Simon & Schuster.

Desrosiers, L., Saint-Jean, M., & Breton, J. (2015). Treatment planning: A key milestone to prevent treatment dropout in adolescents with borderline personality disorder. *Psychology and Psychotherapy: Theory Research and Practice, 88,* 178–196.

Falvey, J. E., Bray, T. E., & Hebert, D. J. (2005). Case conceptualization and treatment planning investigation of problem solving and clinical judgment. *Journal of Mental Health Counseling, 27*(4), 348–372.

Gazzillo, F., Dimaggio, G., & Curtis, J. T. (2021). Case formulation and treatment planning: How to take care of relationship and symptoms together. *Journal of Psychotherapy Integration, 31*(2), 115–128.

Gopi, G., Preeti, S., Ameen, S., & Gowda, M. (2019). Newer documentary practices as per Mental Healthcare Act 2017. *Indian Journal of Psychiatry, 61,* 686-692.

Gutierrez, D., Fox, J., Jones, K., & Fallon, E. (2018). The treatment planning of experienced counselors: A qualitative examination. *Journal of Counseling & Development, 96,* 86–96.

Hatchett, G. T. (2020). Anticipating and planning for the duration of counseling. *Journal of Mental Health Counseling, 42,* 1–14.

Hoffman, B. M., & Meier, S. T. (2001). An individualized approach to managed health mental health care in colleges and universities: A case study. *Journal of College Student Psychotherapy, 15*(4), 49–63.

Kelly, A. (2023, April 27). *Behavioral health treatment plans.* Courtemanche & Associates. https://www.courtemanche-assocs.com/blogs/behavioral-health-treatment-plans

Lee, K. P. (2010). Planning for success: Setting SMART goals for study. *British Journal of Midwifery, 18*(11), 744–746.

Myers, J. E., Sweeney, T. J., & Witmer, J. M. (2000). The wheel of wellness counseling for wellness: A holistic model for treatment planning. *Journal of Counseling & Development, 78,* 251–266.

National Alliance on Mental Illness. (n.d.). *Understanding your diagnosis.* Retrieved January 28, 2024, from https://www.nami.org/your-journey/individuals-with-mental-illness/understanding-your-diagnosis/

National Association of Social Workers. (2021). *Code of ethics of the National Association of Social Workers.* https://www.socialworkers.org/About/Ethics/Code-of-Ethics/Code-of-Ethics

National Board for Certified Counselors. (2023). *NBCC code of ethics.*

Pham, A. P., Berman, J. S., & Lewin, R. K. (2019). Does involving patients in treatment decisions affect perceptions of treatments and therapists? *Society for Psychotherapy Research, 30*(4), 487–494.

Piazza, N. J., & Baruth, N. E. (1990). In the field: Client record guidelines. *Journal of Counseling & Development, 68,* 313–316.

Restifo, S. (2011). Beyond diagnosis- and therapy-centered therapy: The case for incorporating contextual factors in psychotherapy treatment planning. *Australian Psychiatry, 19*(4), 309–312.

Seligman, L. (1993). *Teaching treatment planning.* https://web.p.ebscohost.com/ehost/detail/detail?vid=24&sid=2d8a...eXBIPWEwLHNoaWlmc210ZT1aG9zdC1saXZl#AN=1993-47040-001@db=psych

Shapiro, J. P. (2009). Integrating outcome research and clinical reasoning in psychotherapy planning. *Professional Psychology: Research and Practice, 40*(1), 46–53.

Wiger, D. E. (2012). *The psychotherapy documentation primer* (3rd ed.). John Wiley & Sons.

Wubbolding, R. E., Casstevens, W. J., & Fulkerson, M. H. (2017). Using the WDEP system of reality therapy to support person-centered treatment planning. *Journal of Counseling & Development, 95,* 472–477.

CHAPTER 8

Case Notes

Mona Gallo, EdD, and Gregory L. Bohner, PhD

INTRODUCTION

No matter the mental health discipline or a practitioner's theoretical orientation, clinicians are generally required to generate a case note following any clinical engagement with a client (even a benign phone call regarding scheduling). Case notes are often the central part of most clinical records because they are the record of regular clinical engagement between a provider and the client, document treatment progress or lack thereof, provide clinical insights into the client's patterns and themes, the diagnosis, and the verified rationale for the diagnosis, and provide records of testing and assessments, as well as the plan for treatment. Case notes not only provide a record of clinical engagement and stimulate the review of the course of treatment but also may be a mechanism of communication used between providers, accrediting bodies, and third-party payers, stimulate the review of the course of treatment, and are a legal record and part of the client's protected health information (Baird, 2005; Erford, 2015; Piazza & Baruth, 1990). Documenting all clinical interactions may sometimes seem burdensome and only a part of an administrative process. However, if notes are not documented clearly and succinctly, it may create an ethical or legal risk for the therapist (Raggi et al., 2008; Zhang & Parsons, 2016).

There are several objectives in writing case notes. Case notes need to be clear, brief, and precise while still recording all the vital information. At times, this may be challenging given some case notes programs only provide a limited documentation space and often a limited time frame in which to complete them (Baird, 2005). Baird's (2005) advice for writing case notes is to document the events of the session with the following questions in mind: Will you be able to know what you documented after some time elapses, and will other providers, auditors, or third-party payers be able to track the data documented? If the primary clinician is unavailable to provide support to the client, well-documented case notes increase the chances that another provider will be able to provide relevant assistance (Hutchinson et al., 2008). Another suggestion to clinicians writing case notes is to verify the details in the case note are clear to the clinician and others reviewing the case note but also vague enough to protect the client if the documentation was to be subpoenaed. Clinicians should document the details in the case note in an accurate and precise way to protect themselves if the documentation was to be used in a legal proceeding against the clinician.

There are multiple purposes in documenting a case note. The predominant purpose in writing a case note is to improve and enhance the treatment process by assisting the clinician and other treating professionals in tracking the client's progress in treatment while staying focused on the treatment plan. Case notes should document the goal of the therapeutic session. This goal needs to reflect the treatment plan and optimally connect one session to the next. The goal does not need to be so rigid that it is what directs the therapeutic session, but it should be flexible enough to address any acute client concerns that may be presented in a session. It is best that a case note includes the assessment of the clinician's therapeutic technique(s) or intervention(s). This assessment should also include what technique(s) and intervention(s) worked and what could be improved upon. It is also important to include an objective clinical impression of the client based on client statements or behavior. It is necessary to review the clinical impression and test it for subjectivity. Clinicians should avoid documenting untested or subjective clinical impressions in client documentation. Do not use language that could be deemed disparaging by the client. A good practice is to write case notes as if the client will be reading them at some point. Clinicians' opinions should be backed by information obtained from the client, theory, or relevant literature. Avoid the use of abbreviations that are not an established practice within the field and extraneous information that is not pertinent to client treatment (McCulloch, 2023). Lastly, case notes should also contain a plan of action that can demonstrate clinician thoughtfulness in the client's treatment, as well as a continuity of care from session to session (Piazza & Baruth, 1990).

Documenting a clinical case note can be easier and more accurate when generated directly following the clinician–client engagement. Clinicians should earmark enough time to generate timely and accurate clinical documentation (Erford, 2015). If a clinician waits until lunch time, the end of the day, or even the next day, the possibility of cross-transferring and confusing information from one client case to another increases. Specific and crucial details may also be forgotten, as memory decays across time (Falvey et al., 2005; Zhang & Parsons, 2016). Outside of confusion and memory decay, if the clinician leaves the clinical notes unaddressed until some later time, something may happen to the clinical clinician or facility that inhibits completing the case note or completely prohibits them from documenting at all (i.e., accident, emergency health situation, something happens at or to the facility). Timely and accurate client case notes also support the clinician in building a higher level of care for each client and reducing potential specific ethical and legal risks for the clinician (Zhang & Parsons, 2016).

To Quote or Not to Quote

According to Cameron and turtle-song (2002), there are multiple reasons clinicians should use quotations in case notes sparingly and judiciously. The clinician should avoid direct quotations that specifically identify other people by name and sometimes by title (i.e., dad, mom, aunt, etc.) and provocative statements related to other providers because these other providers may be accessing the case note as part of a treatment team. This could hamper or impede upon comprehensive and impartial client care. An overuse of quotations may make it difficult for providers to distinguish client themes and monitor the efficacy of clinical interventions. When reviewed by any outside entity, the accuracy or integrity of the case note could be subject to scrutiny because verbatim quotations are often difficult to recall after just a minute or so, let alone after a full-length counseling session. It is not to say that quotations used in case notes cannot be accurate or even beneficial, but Cameron and turtle-song (2002) suggest that clinicians only quote key words or brief phrases that the client shares and only in instances where the data would be crucial (i.e., threats to the self or others, aggressive comments toward clinician, difficulty in orientation, confusion, increased efficacy due to treatment successes, etc.).

Whether the clinician is quoting exactly what the client said or documenting the general idea of what the client said, it is imperative that the clinician indicates the client's sharing with language that is clear enough for any reader to distinguish. Some words that indicate that the data documented came directly from the client are "stated," "reported," "shared," "commented," "complained," "disclosed," and so on. Clinicians need to clearly differentiate what the client shares and what is observed. If the clinician is observing themes, patterns, behaviors, affect, and the like, then the data documented needs to clearly indicate the observation through words such as "saw," "observed," "noticed," "perceived," "detected," and so on. If the clinician is not necessarily clear on what has been observed, then the clinician can document data with words such as "appeared" or "seemed." However, in instances where the clinician is unsure and hypothesizing in the written documentation, the clinician should follow up with the evidence that leads them to the presumption. Here is a brief example: "The client appeared down and sullen by evidence of their slumped posture and inability to maintain eye contact, which is different from the history of clinical engagement. Client was unkempt, lacking typical grooming, by history. Client denied being depressed."

Theory in Case Notes

Although not generally mandated by employers or third-party payers, it can be tremendously important for the clinician to document their use of theory and how it guides a client's treatment in the case note. When incorporating the use of theory into case notes, the clinician would use theory-congruent language and document the view of the client from the theoretical lens that informs the clinician's treatment approach. Remember, this view needs to remain objective, not subjective (Piazza & Baruth, 1990). The use of theoretical language will appear in the data that documents the clinical impression of the client and their problems, sometimes in the assessments used, as well as the interpretation of the results of the assessment or the plan of treatment, and possibly for the choice of adjunct treatment or treatment providers.

ETHICAL NEED FOR DOCUMENTING IN CASE NOTES

Even though case notes are regularly reviewed by outside bodies such as third-party payers or auditing companies, it is best for clinicians to remember the ethical and legal implications when completing clinician documentation and let the concerns related to third-party reimbursement be secondary concerns. It is necessary for a clinician to refer to and follow their own professional code of ethics when documenting client care, including case notes.

Although the American Counseling Association ([ACA], 2014), the American Psychological Association ([APA], 2017), and the National Association of Social Workers ([NASW], 2021) do not explicitly address case note documentation within their ethical codes, there are guidelines regarding documentation that clinicians need to astutely follow. All three professional associations—ACA, APA, and NASW—stress the need for the clinician to implement reasonable precautions in protecting the client's confidential information, which includes case notes.

Clinicians keep clinical notes to assist in rendering services. Clinicians are guided to release clinical data to third-party payers when there has been authorization and disclose with consent unless legally mandated. Mentioned previously, the *2014 ACA Code of Ethics* (ACA, 2014) also directs the retention, transfer, and destruction of records. The code advises clinicians to guard the transferring of case notes, whether for continuity of care or third-party payment. Notes are to be kept secure, no matter how stored (ACA, 2014).

In the *Ethical Principles of Psychologists and Code of Conduct* (APA, 2017), disclosure is limited to the minimum necessary to obtain payment. This implies that the information in a case note is vaguely specific—vague enough to protect the client or others in the client's life and specific enough to protect the clinician. As mentioned in previous chapters, this code of conduct also governs the retention, distribution, and destruction of records: Records are to be accurate and need to be compliant with the state and federal laws (APA, 2017).

In the *Code of Ethics of the National Association of Social Workers* (NASW, 2021), clinicians are directed to document clinical data accurately and in a timely fashion to reflect services, facilitate the delivery of services, and provide a continuity of care. This code of ethics emphasizes documenting data that reflects only the services provided; again, the wording lends itself to the documentation needing to be vaguely specific. As mentioned in previous chapters, the *NASW (2021) code* also directs the clinician in retention, transfer, and destruction of records, which includes case notes.

LEGAL NEED FOR DOCUMENTING IN CASE NOTES

Most states have statutes and regulations that require clinicians to maintain client clinical documentation. Maintaining current client documentation is an important part of a clinician providing beneficial services to clients, recording that relevant services were delivered, and furnishing the opportunity for a continuity of care to clients in the absence of the original clinician or in conjunction with adjunct providers (Erford, 2015).

When considering legal ramifications, clinicians should be cautious regarding what they put in their progress notes. Take care to review before submitting an official progress note to ensure there are not any words suggesting bias or prejudice. Also, confirm there are not any conclusions noted, such as a diagnosis, without substantial justification. It would be wise for clinicians to immediately correct any errors in a client's file as soon as possible. A line should be struck through the error with the clinician noting the date and signing initials next to the correction (Hartsell & Bernstein, 2008). Being thorough in all documentation may help avoid problematic issues in the future.

Unlike progress notes, which are part of the client's private health information and therefore subject to being disclosed upon specific allowable requests by the client and/or other parties in legal proceedings, psychotherapy notes are not considered part of the designated record set required for each client. According to the HIPAA Privacy Rule (Standards for Privacy of Individually Identifiable Health Information, 2000), they are separate notes kept by the clinician that are used to document or analyze the discussions during therapy sessions. Psychotherapy notes would exclude information related to medication and prescription monitoring, clinical assessment results, start and end time of sessions, therapeutic modality utilized, frequency of sessions, diagnosis, mental health status, symptoms, prognosis, progress, or treatment plan. These details are all part of the client's medical record and subject to disclosure when legally required. However, to ensure proper protocol, psychotherapy notes should be kept in a file separate from the client's designated record set.

INSURANCE PURPOSES FOR DOCUMENTING IN CASE NOTES

Most third-party payers expect to see several pieces of documentation as a part of their reimbursement process. In general, third-party payers want evidence for the need of counseling through a diagnosis (justifying services), a plan for treatment (treatment plan), and documentation that indicates services were provided to the client and that the client is progressing through their treatment (case notes), and when treatment ends, third-party payers want to know that the services have ended (discharge/termination summary). Without appropriate and thorough documentation, clients may be denied services and/or the clinician may be denied reimbursement.

INFORMATION TO INCLUDE IN THE CASE NOTE

Budding and sometimes seasoned clinicians can feel overwhelmed and confused when deciding what data to include or exclude in case notes. Common questions include: What data do I need to include? What data do I need to leave out? How do I document enough data to protect myself, ethically and legally? What do I leave out to protect the client, ethically and legally? Do I document in third person or first person? What data goes where? How do I state data? Do I quote? How much do I quote? If I have a choice, what note style do I use? How do I document the theoretical orientation in the note? Many of these questions can be answered through education, exposure, and practice (Prieto & Scheel, 2002; Sperry, 2005).

Since clinical documentation is generally occurring after the clinical encounter with the client, it is best to use past-tense language in the case note. This is unless the client has agreed to do something such as complete homework, practice a skill, take an initiative, or attend a referral in between sessions. Then the clinician would document that "The client has agreed to ..." or "The client stated they will ..." using future-tense language. The clinician needs to be mindful of what tense they are using in the language depicted in clinical documentation, as this denotes if the client has done or is going to fulfill what they are accounting for in the documentation.

No matter the case note format the clinician chooses, there is essential data that should appear in every case note. Many authors have different ideas as to what data should appear in a case note. The following list may not include all considerations but is a relatively comprehensive list of considerations for a clinician:

- The clinician should include any discussions or references to the client's informed consent.
- Each case note needs to include objectives and goals worked towards in session, client symptoms, the diagnosis(es), and any differential diagnoses.

- The clinician should consider including the client's presenting problem, the client's presentation and functional status observed by the clinician, and engagement or lack thereof with the clinician and treatment.
- The clinician should document the interventions they used during the appointment and the client's response to the interventions, along with any interventions the client has or will use outside of direct treatment.
- The clinician should include any emergency-related reports, such as the client being a danger to the self or others, reported abuse or neglect, and, in some states, reported domestic or intimate partner violence.
- If any assessments/tests were provided, the clinician would document the name of the instrument utilized, the client's score/results, as well as the clinical interpretation of the assessment results and prognosis of the client.
- It is best for the clinician to document any referrals, even to informal engagements (i.e., book club, hiking group, National Alliance on Mental Illness), and the date and time of the next scheduled appointment. (Hutchinson et al., 2008; Zhang & Parsons, 2016.)

Language to Use in the Case Note

Case notes may be read by treatment team members, the client, third-party payers, stakeholders, or other professionals. Therefore, clinicians are encouraged to use professional and clinical language that is void of jargon, colloquialism, or words that may be misunderstood. Clinicians are encouraged to remember they are writing to anyone who may read the clinical documentation, not just for their own professional reference.

By Report

Generally, the language used within case notes that indicates that the client is sharing information will appear written using phrases such as "The client reported ..." or "The client stated ..." The clinician can use quotes here, but it is also sufficient to just paraphrase what the client said to the clinician about how they felt, thought, or experienced the data they shared.

By Observation

The language used within case notes will generally be written from the clinician's voice, third person, and regarding the observations of the client within the clinical context. The clinician can use language such as "The clinician observed ..." "The client appeared ... by evidence of ..." or "The client seemed ... by evidence of ..." for clarity.

Theoretical Reference

In case notes, documenting the client's objectives worked on and the clinical interventions from a theoretical perspective can support the clinician's use of evidence-based practices. The reference to the use of theory can help guide the client's treatment and should be included in case notes.

Clinical Intervention

Clinical interventions are creative tools and techniques, often directly related to theory-specific treatment, that the clinician will or has used to assist the client in making treatment progress (Hutchinson et al., 2008). The documentation of the action steps related to clinical interventions should record what the client is and will be working on, as well as what the client has achieved thus far. The use of clinical interventions to help the client meet their objectives and overall goals is imperative in treatment.

Plan

The plan section of a case note should include, at a minimum, three key pieces of information. These items are the date and time of the next scheduled appointment, what homework the client agrees to complete in between their appointments, and any relevant referrals.

DATE/TIME

The date and time may appear twice in a case note. The clinician needs to document the date of the appointment that the case note reflects. It is best practice that the clinician documents the date and time of the next scheduled appointment as well. This future date can be documented in the plan section of a case note, such as "The client scheduled their next appointment for (date) and (time)." In some cases, the client does not know their upcoming schedule and will have to contact the clinician for their next appointment. In this case, the clinician can document an unscheduled appointment by writing, "The client will contact the clinician for their next appointment due to not knowing their schedule." There are times the client is doing well and wants to wait to schedule their next appointment based on trying to live independently without regular counseling contact. In this case, the clinician can document, "The client will return as needed."

HOMEWORK

The reference to homework may appear in two sections of a case note. Near the beginning of the case note, it may be noted that the client and/or clinician has followed up on what the client agreed to do in between sessions, even if it is not "formal" homework like a worksheet but just a skill practiced, such as "exercised three times since last session."

Also note the client's interpretation of how they or others were impacted by what they agreed to perform or practice in between appointments. This denotation of homework would be stated in past tense, as it would have already been completed.

The other place homework may appear is in the plan section of the case note. In this section, the clinician is documenting what the client agrees to do, perform, or practice in between the two appointments. The language here would be in future tense, denoting what the client will be doing.

REFERRALS

It is imperative to connect clients with other relevant outside sources. The referral section of a case note is intended to demonstrate the clinician's attempt to connect a client to any outside services or supports. Referrals can be formal or informal. Examples of formal referrals include case management, medical, dental, or a treatment facility. Examples of informal referrals include Alcoholics Anonymous, the senior center, or an activity group at school. Connecting the client with resources, support, healthy ways for clients to express themselves, and the like is wise, and it also wise to document you did so in the plan section of case notes.

SOAP NOTES

One of the most frequently used case note styles is the SOAP note. The SOAP acronym stands for subjective (S), objective (O), assessment (A), plan (P). The SOAP note style was developed in the mid-1960s by Lawrence L. Weed to address problem-oriented medical records (Weed, 1968; Zhang & Parsons, 2016).

The subjective (S) section of the SOAP case note is what the client or other stakeholders report. This section also includes what the client reports regarding their thoughts, feelings, plans, goals, and actions and how the client believes things are positively or negatively affecting their life. The subjective section may include client statements in quotes, but it is not required. Either way, use action words, such as "The client stated, reported, acknowledged, refuted, denied, expressed, shared, clarified, conveyed, and so on," in the subjective section to indicate the client's actual report, which differentiates the data from any observations (Cameron & turtle-song, 2002; Zhang & Parsons, 2016).

The objective (O) section of this case note style of case note is where factual data is reported. This data can include the clinician's observations of the client's appearance, affect, behaviors, orientation, relationship with the clinician, any strengths or weaknesses, responses to treatment, medication compliance or lack thereof, and any other clinical provider's observations. The data recorded in this section remains evidence-based and free from opinion, judgment, or imposition of the clinician's values. The language used needs to be exact and descriptive. If a clinician decides to use interpretive wording such as "seems" or "appears," then a justification of evidence needs to be provided in conjunction with the observations. The objective section should include language that clearly differentiates the clinician's observations from client statements. Use action phrases such as "The clinician observed ..." and/or "By evidence of ..." when documenting direction observations (Cameron & turtle-song, 2002; Zhang & Parsons, 2016).

The assessment (A) section of the SOAP case note must be based on the combination and interpretation of the subjective and objective data. The clinician would also include their clinical impressions, as well as the diagnosis and the differential diagnosis(es). If the clinician is unsure of the final diagnosis, then include a provisional diagnosis. Whether there is a substantiated final diagnosis is present in this section or a provisional diagnosis, the summary data from the (S) and (O) sections should support the indicated diagnosis. In addition, the assessment section is an excellent place to include the client's prognosis and supporting reasons for the prognosis (Cameron & turtle-song, 2002; Zhang & Parsons, 2016).

When documenting the plan (P) section of the SOAP case note, it is best practice to include the date and time of the next scheduled appointment. Clinicians will want to document any interventions utilized during the current session, as well as any interventions or homework the client agreed to use in between the current and coming appointment. Clinicians may also document any interventions that the client may be utilizing while working with other providers. Data documented in the plan section may also include treatment progress and any changes to treatment, as well as any consultation regarding the client's treatment. And lastly, it is best practice to include some kind of referral. Referrals do not have to be formal referrals, such as to a psychiatrist or group counseling, but could include referrals to outside social groups or to some type of community engagement. If the referral is to a formal provider, then it is important for the clinician to document the name and contact information of the direct referral (Cameron & turtle-song, 2002; Zhang & Parsons, 2016).

SECTION OF SOAP CASE NOTE	WHAT IS INCLUDED IN THE SECTION
SUBJECTIVE (S)	What the client reports (i.e., thoughts, feelings, goals, plans, actions) and the client's impressions regarding the intensity of the concerns and the impact on relationships What stakeholders report about the client (i.e., family members, teachers, case managers, etc.) Descriptions of how the client experiences their world (i.e., impressions on how change is affecting them, relationships, or their environment)

OBJECTIVE (O)	Factual information that the clinician observes (i.e., client affect, appearance, behavior, orientation x4, strengths, weaknesses) The clinician's interpretation of the counseling relationship (i.e., client's engagement or lack thereof)
ASSESSMENT (A)	Summary of the clinician's clinical thinking (i.e., clinical diagnosis, differential diagnosis, clinical impressions) Combined interpretation of the subjective and objective data (i.e., clinical impressions, labeling of the client's behavior, and hypothesis of the reason behind the behavior) The client's prognosis (i.e., poor, guarded, fair, good, excellent) Any testing results obtained by the clinician or from other providers, which should be included in the client file
PLAN (P)	Date and time of the next scheduled appointment A description of the treatment (i.e., interventions utilized, any treatment progress and direction, plans to changes in treatment and the rationale) Any activities to be performed in between appointments (i.e., homework, other treatment providers, activities, agreed-upon plans) Any referrals (i.e., medical professionals, adjunct providers, engagement in community or social activities, etc.)

DAP NOTES

Another frequently utilized case note style is the DAP note. The DAP acronym stands for data/description (D), assessment/analysis (A), and plan (P). This case note style is the second most frequently used case note style, but it is gaining popularity due to its ease of use.

The data (D) section of the DAP case note format is like the combination of the subjective and objective sections from the SOAP note format; however, it remains more grounded in the factual content retrieved during the client's session. This section can include client or clinician statements in quotes, but the language used needs to differentiate between what the client reported or stated and what the clinician stated. The data section will also include information related to the client's thoughts, feelings, plans, goals, actions, and how the client's life and/or relationships are positively or negatively affected. If the clinician is observing data documented, then the language used needs to clearly indicate it is a clinical observation. This section can include data from stakeholders. The clinician is encouraged to document their clinical impression, which may include a description of the client's appearance, affect, mood, behaviors, and speech. The (D) section of the DAP case note format may also include any objectives addressed during the session, interventions utilized, review of the treatment plan, review of any homework or referrals from previous appointments, and if any consultation was obtained (Zhang & Parsons, 2016).

In the assessment (A) section of the DAP case note format, the clinician would document their interpretation of the client's problem, along with their hypothesis of the client's concerns. This hypothesis can include the clinician's understanding of the underlying patterns or issues that may be the cause of or exasperating the client's presenting problem. This section needs to include the client's diagnosis and differential diagnosis(es). Again, if a diagnosis has not been determined, then it is best to utilize a provisional diagnosis. If any testing or assessments have been used, including a mental status exam, then the results and interpretations would be included in this section of the DAP case note. In the assessment section, the clinician would document the client's current response to treatment, any progress or lack thereof, and how the current session supports the client's overall treatment (Zhang & Parsons, 2016).

In the plan (P) section of the DAP case note format, the clinician should document the date and time of the next scheduled appointment. Clinicians will want to document any revisions to the client's treatment plan, any agreed-upon interventions or homework that the client will accomplish between appointments, as well as the client's engagement with adjunct providers or interventions from other providers. Lastly, the plan section is concluded with a referral. Again, referrals do not need to be to formal providers but can be related to social or community engagements (i.e., community center, senior center, meetup group, etc.). But if a referral to another provider is furnished, then the name and contact information should be documented (Cameron & turtle-song, 2002; Zhang & Parsons, 2016).

SECTION OF DAP CASE NOTE	WHAT IS INCLUDED IN THE SECTION
DATA/ DESCRIPTION (D)	What the client reports (i.e., thoughts, feelings, goals, plans, actions) and the client's impressions regarding the intensity of the concerns and the impact on relationships What stakeholders report about the client (i.e., family members, teachers, case managers, etc.) Descriptions of how the client experiences their world (i.e., orientation x4, impressions on how change is affecting them, relationships, or their environment) Factual information that the clinician observes (i.e., client affect, appearance, behavior, strengths, weaknesses) The clinician's interpretation of the counseling relationship (i.e., client's engagement or lack thereof) Review (i.e., homework, other provider engagement, follow-up on referral appointments)

ASSESSMENT/ ANALYSIS (A)	Summary of the clinician's clinical thinking (i.e., clinical diagnosis, differential diagnosis, clinical impressions) Combined interpretation of the subjective and objective data (i.e., clinical impressions, labeling of the client's behavior, and hypothesis of the reason behind the behavior) Review (i.e., client's responses to treatment, any testing results from other providers that would be including the client file)
PLAN (P)	Date and time of the next scheduled appointment A description of the treatment (i.e., interventions utilized, any treatment progress and direction, plans to changes in treatment and the rationale) The client's prognosis (i.e., poor, poor, guarded, fair, good, excellent) Any activities to be performed in between appointments (i.e., homework, other treatment providers, activities, agreed-upon plans) Any referrals (i.e., medical professionals, adjunct providers, engagement in community or social activities, etc.)

DART NOTES

The DART acronym stands for description (D), assessment (A), response (R), and treatment (T). This case note style was developed for mental health professionals in the early 2000s by Brian N. Baird (Zhang & Parsons, 2016). Baird's (2005) DART note format can prompt a clinician to document what happened, what the clinician's interpretation was, how the clinician responded, and what the clinician believes they and the client should do in the immediate future.

The description (D) section of this style of case note is developed through a description of answering the questions "When?" "Where?" "Who?" and "What?" The "when" is the date and time. The "where" should document the location, unless it is the same location consistently (Baird, 2005). The "who" is the person or people who participated, including who was present with the client when a situation or event occurred (Baird, 2005). And the "what" is the description of what occurred, what was reported by the client in session, or what was observed by the clinician. Arguably, the most malleable piece of the description (D) section is the "what." Documenting what occurred may require more details and dedicated space in the description section (Baird, 2005; Zhang & Parsons, 2016).

The assessment (A) section of this case note style is the space where the clinician would answer the "why." Answering the "why" means documenting what has been observed by the clinician and the clinician's interpretation of the meaning behind these observations. The clinician may consider how the client's current presentation, thinking, or behavior may relate (a) to previous data the clinician has obtained regarding the client, (b) to the client's current situations, (c) to the client's treatment, or (d) to other known factors. A clinician is not necessarily tasked with providing an explanation or interpretation but instead is documenting the observations and noting if the client has deviated from their normal presentation. If a clinician does not immediately understand the meaning behind an observation, then the suggestion is to document the need for further or future consideration (Baird, 2005; Zhang & Parsons, 2016).

The response (R) section is where the clinician documents their response to what has been observed, interpreted, or assessed. Data to document in the response section would be interventions used, assessments or evaluations conducted and their scores, information provided to the client, referrals made, clinical consultations, as well as choices made not to provide a response. The clinician should include the consideration of the risks and benefits of the response, always including the clinician's rationale for the response. It is imperative to use clear, descriptive, and accurate language that indicates the logic for the steps the clinician decided to implement (Baird, 2005; Zhang & Parsons, 2016). The more detailed the response section is, the more it can reduce the questions regarding clinical negligence if a legal query arises (Baird, 2005).

The last section of this case note style is the treatment (T) section. This section is where the clinician will document such things as the next scheduled appointment date and time, the next steps in treatment, any homework, the inclusion of other treatment providers, any referrals, and the rationale for the inclusion of other treatment providers or referrals along with the name and contact information for the direct referral (Baird, 2005; Cameron & turtle-song, 2002; Zhang & Parsons, 2016). Details in the treatment section of this case note need to be specific, detailed enough to protect the clinician, and written clearly enough for other viewers to understand (Baird, 2005; Zhang & Parsons, 2016).

SECTION OF DART CASE NOTE	WHAT IS INCLUDED IN THE SECTION
DESCRIPTION (D)	What the client reports (i.e., thoughts, feelings, goals, plans, actions) and the client's impressions regarding the intensity of the concerns and the impact on relationships What stakeholders report about the client (i.e., family members, teachers, case managers, etc.) Descriptions of how the client experiences their world (i.e., orientation x4, impressions on how change is affecting them, relationships, or their environment) Factual information that the clinician observes (i.e., client affect, appearance, behavior, strengths, weaknesses) Review (i.e., homework, other provider engagement, follow-up on referral appointments)

ASSESSMENT (A)	Summary of the clinician's clinical thinking (i.e., clinical diagnosis, differential diagnosis, clinical impressions) The client's prognosis (i.e., poor, poor, guarded, fair, good, excellent) Review (i.e., client's responses to treatment, any testing results from other providers that would be including the client file)
RESPONSE (R)	The clinician's interpretation of the counseling relationship (i.e., client's engagement or lack thereof) A description of the treatment (i.e., interventions utilized, any treatment progress and direction, plans to changes in treatment and the rationale)
TREATMENT (T)	Date and time of the next scheduled appointment Any activities to be performed in between appointments (i.e., homework, other treatment providers, activities, agreed-upon plans) Any referrals (i.e., medical professionals, adjunct providers, engagement in community or social activities, etc.)

BIRP NOTES

Another widely utilized format of session note taking is the BIRP note. BIRP is an acronym for behavior (B), intervention (I), response (R), and plan (P). This note-taking method is like the other styles already addressed but also differs in a couple of ways. One way the BIRP differs from other note styles is the combination of objective, subjective, and assessment information into the behavior (B) section (Reiter & Sabo, 2023). By doing so, clinicians focus upon combining all notes about behavior into one section rather than having to identify which sections it would be appropriate to assign specific behaviors to. This combination of data includes elements of the client's self-report and clinician's observations. In terms of other note formats, this would be a combination of the subjective, objective, and assessment sections of the SOAP note, the data and assessment sections of the DAP note, and the description and assessment sections of the DART note.

While combining objective, subjective, and assessment information into the behavior (B) section, it remains important for the clinician to be succinct in writing and not allow this section to become bloated with superfluous information. As a reminder, this type of information is more suited for psychotherapy notes and not for progress notes. Therefore, record the behaviors that contribute to the client's presenting problem and how those contribute to the assessment and diagnosis of the client's present condition.

The BIRP note also emphasizes the impacts of utilized interventions as a part of the therapeutic process, which is documented in the intervention (I) section of the BIRP note. While the behavior (B), response (R), and plan (P) sections are primarily concerned with what the client is doing and how that contributes to their current state, the intervention (I) section is focused upon what the clinician is doing as part of the therapeutic process.

Some therapeutic approaches (e.g., cognitive behavioral therapy, solution-focused brief therapy) provide a clear view of which interventions were used in session and how well the client has responded to the interventions. No matter the theory used, clinicians should document information such as specific techniques or questions that were asked in the session in the intervention (I) section of a BIRP note (Reiter & Sabo, 2023). While listing interventions in a bulleted list may be sufficient in some cases, clinicians may also consider adding brief sentences demonstrating questions used or feedback provided to the client.

In the response (R) section of a BIRP note, the clinician would document the outcome of the client experiencing the intervention. While this often includes the client's immediate in-session reactions, both verbal and behavioral (Reiter & Sabo, 2023), this space also allows the clinician to track client experiences utilizing interventions outside of the therapy session. For example, in a fourth session with a client, the clinician may document that they taught the client how to engage in box breathing exercises in the intervention (I) section of the note. They would then briefly describe how well the client performed the activity and the client's affective response to utilizing box breathing in the response section. In the fifth session, the clinician will follow up with the client about the use of the intervention and gather information about how well it impacted the client's symptoms outside of session. This additional information in the fifth session can also be recorded in the response (R) section even though the introduction of the intervention occurred in the fourth session.

Finally, the plan (P) section of a BIRP note will appear familiar, as it is set up in the same manner as the plan section of the SOAP and DAP notes. Clinicians will document data such as the next scheduled session or rationale for not scheduling a new appointment, any homework the client has decided to accomplish between sessions, any referrals, and the current prognosis of the client. As appropriate, therapists should reference the treatment plan and goals of therapy as part of the long-term planning for therapy.

SECTION OF BIRP CASE NOTE	WHAT IS INCLUDED IN THE SECTION
BEHAVIOR (B)	What the client reports (i.e., thoughts, feelings, goals, plans, actions) and the client's impressions regarding the intensity of the concerns and the impact on relationships What stakeholders report about the client (i.e., family members, teachers, case managers, etc.) Descriptions of how the client experiences their world (i.e., orientation x4, impressions on how change is affecting them, relationships, or their environment)

	Factual information that the clinician observes (i.e., client affect, appearance, behavior, strengths, weaknesses) Summary of the clinician's clinical thinking (i.e., clinical diagnosis, differential diagnosis, clinical impressions) Review (i.e., homework, other provider engagement, follow-up on referral appointments)
INTERVENTION (I)	A description of the treatment (i.e., interventions utilized and the client's response, any treatment progress and direction, plans to changes in treatment and the rationale)
RESPONSE (R)	A description of the client's behavioral and verbal responses to treatment (i.e., interventions utilized, any treatment progress and direction, plans to changes in treatment and the rationale) in session. Review (i.e., client's responses to treatment outside of session, any testing results from other providers that would be including the client file)
PLAN (P)	Date and time of the next scheduled appointment The client's prognosis (i.e., poor, poor, guarded, fair, good, excellent) Any activities to be performed in between appointments (i.e., homework, other treatment providers, activities, agreed-upon plans) Any referrals (i.e., medical professionals, adjunct providers, engagement in community or social activities, etc.)

PI-DIB NOTES

The PI-DIB case note style was developed and researched by a team of licensed clinicians who wanted to generate a clinical note that would represent the mental health field more accurately than the traditional medical case notes (SOAP, DAP, BIRP) that clinicians have used for decades. The PI-DIB case note style represents the process of conceptualizing a client's case through the five sections represented in the PI-DIB format (Dubi et al., 2012; Raggi et al., 2008).

The PI-DIB acronym stands for problem (P), issues (I), dynamic (D), interventions (I), and bridge (B). The problem (P) section is where the clinician documents their understanding of the client's presenting problem by means of what the client reports and through the clinician's theoretical understanding. The issue (I) section is where the clinician documents the underlying issues of the client that may be reframed by the clinician. The client may have underlying issues related to safety, fear, self-esteem, self-efficacy, control, choices, self-talk, and so on. Extending the conceptualization of the client's presenting problem (P) through identifying the underlying issues (I) may accelerate the process of conceptualizing the client's case, which may assist both the client and clinician in more quickly focusing on the deeper sources and concerns of the client.

The dynamic (D) section is distinctive to this case note format and is where the clinician will document the nature of the therapeutic alliance. Decades of research indicate that the distinct characteristics of the client–clinician relationship has a profound effect on the course of treatment (Flückiger et al., 2020; Lambert, 2004). When a clinician examines the therapeutic alliance (i.e., dynamic) following each clinical encounter, this can provoke the clinician to consider how they are engaging with the client and how this may have contributed or failed to contribute to the client's treatment.

The intervention (the second "I" section) is where the clinician further conceptualizes the client's case by assessing the interventions proposed or used and how they relate to the client's presenting problems and issues. This section can assist the clinician in expeditiously assessing the suitability and efficacy of the intervention.

The last section of this case note style is the bridge (B) between sessions, and this section prompts the clinician to examine the close of the session. The clinician would document their observations, client expectations for the next session, as well as any commitments the client made that would occur in between sessions (i.e., homework, follow-up with referrals, attending appointments with adjunct treatment providers; Dubi et al., 2012; Raggi et al., 2008). If a direct referral to an adjunct provider is supplied to the client, then the name and contact information of the referral needs to be documented (Cameron & turtle-song, 2002).

Although a newer and less known format, the PI-DIB case note provides a straightforward framework for clinicians to utilize. Scant research on this style of case note demonstrated clinicians found that using the PI-DIB style note assisted them and supervised trainees in conceptualizing the client's case more deeply, as well as thinking critically about the client's presenting problem and the issues underlying the problem. It was also reported that this case note style prompted clinicians to examine their practice with the client, as well as how the therapeutic presentation of the clinician impacted the client engagement (Raggi et al., 2008). Naturally, a clinician's professional self-reflection and self-examination can lead to better clinical engagement.

SECTION OF PI-DIB CASE NOTE	WHAT IS INCLUDED IN THE SECTION
PROBLEM (P)	What the client reports (i.e., thoughts, feelings, goals, plans, actions) and the client's impressions regarding the intensity of the concerns and the impact on relationships What stakeholders report about the client (i.e., family members, teachers, case managers, etc.) Factual information that the clinician observes (i.e., client affect, appearance, behavior, strengths, weaknesses) Review (i.e., homework, other provider engagement, follow-up on referral appointments)

ISSUE (I)	Descriptions of how the client experiences their world (i.e., orientation x4, impressions on how change is affecting them, relationships, or their environment) Summary of the clinician's clinical thinking (i.e., clinical diagnosis, differential diagnosis, clinical impressions) The client's prognosis (i.e., poor, guarded, fair, good, excellent)
DYNAMIC (D)	The clinician's interpretation of the counseling relationship (i.e., client's engagement or lack thereof) Review (i.e., client's responses to treatment, any testing results from other providers that would be including the client file)
INTERVENTION (2ND I)	A description of the treatment (i.e., interventions utilized, any treatment progress and direction, plans to changes in treatment and the rationale)
BRIDGE (B)	Date and time of the next scheduled appointment Any activities to be performed in between appointments (i.e., homework, other treatment providers, activities, agreed-upon plans) Any referrals (i.e., medical professionals, adjunct providers, engagement in community or social activities, etc.)

NARRATIVE NOTES

Along with other case note styles, narrative case notes tell the story of the treatment episode. Narrative case notes are written in a format that documents the "story" of the client's and clinician's interaction. As with any story, the clinician must provide enough detail that the client is depicted as a unique individual and it is clear how they are engaged in their own treatment process (Hutchinson et al., 2008).

Narrative case notes are frequently written in a format that documents the client's own words and responses to the clinical interaction and the counselor's engagement and interventions. Quotes are often used, documenting what the client or clinician stated during the counseling session. Oftentimes, clinicians who use a narrative case note format will take notes during the counseling session so the details of the engagement are not forgotten and can be accurately documented.

There can be several challenges in using a narrative style case note. One limitation is that relevant data can become buried in the narrative because this note style lacks structure of other note styles that lend themselves to guiding the author, as well as the reader. Another limitation is that the author of a narrative note can add too much irrelevant data that can compromise a level of protection for the client, especially if documentation becomes viewable and scrutinized by people outside of the mental health profession. Additionally, the lack of format while utilizing a narrative case note style may lead the clinician to veer away from including crucial clinical data that support third-party reimbursement and justification for the client's services.

CONCLUSION

Overall, case note formats are very similar in style, with each having a space for clinicians to report clinical data from the client's view and from the clinician's view, with the inclusion of clinical impressions, testing or assessments and their results, as well as documenting what the plan of treatment has and will be. And no matter the case note style chosen, it is imperative that the clinician sign and date the case note and place it in the client's file.

Do not fret, as the skills required to write succinct, clear, and brief case notes, in a short time frame, following any case note format, may be strengthened and mastered by studying applied examples and problem-solving through practiced case note documentation (Kodweis et al., 2021; Prieto & Scheel, 2002).

SOAP NOTE INSTRUCTIONS

Client Name: XXXXXX
Session Date: February 12, 2XXX
Session Number: X

	Type of Session:		Nature of Contact:
	Individual		Scheduled Appointment
	Group		Walk-in
	Couples		Emergency
	Family		

Subjective

Based on the SOAP format, the subjective section should provide information about what happened during the session, including client-reported information (such as presenting problem or symptoms), client's report of suicidal ideation/homicidal ideation (SI/HI) and substance use information, the topics of discussion and their sequence, the client's reported reactions, interventions used, and any discussion related to homework.

Enough information should be provided so that another professional (including your supervisor) can follow exactly what happened during the session. Remember, if it isn't documented, it didn't happen, which can have important implications in terms of liability when others evaluate the quality and thoroughness of the services provided.

Objective

Based on the SOAP format, the objective section should provide the counselor's clinical impressions from the session, including the interpretation of counselor-observed behaviors and emotions (including mental status info.) and a conceptualization of the client's issues (which may align/contrast with client's view/insight).

Assessment

Provide the ICD-10 #, diagnosis and differential diagnosis(es) with specifiers (including any provisional considerations), prognosis, evaluation of SI/HI risk, and any testing results.

Plan

Any plans or recommendations relating to the future of treatment are stated, including the next session's appointment date and time, any referrals, and homework assignments agreed to be completed. Items listed here were either already discussed in session or, if not critical, will happen at or before the very next session.

_______________________ _______________________

(Clinician, Degree, Date) (Supervisor, Degree, Date)

DAP NOTE INSTRUCTIONS

Client Name: XXXXXX
Session Date: February 12, 2XXX
Session Number: X

	Type of Session:		Nature of Contact:
	Individual		Scheduled Appointment
	Group		Walk-in
	Couples		Emergency
	Family		

Data

Based on the DAP format, the data section should provide information about what happened during the session, including client-reported information (such as presenting problem or symptoms), client's report of SI/HI and substance use information, counselor-observed behaviors and emotions, the topics of discussion and their sequence, the client's reported reactions, interventions used, and any discussion related to homework.

Enough information should be provided so that another professional (including your supervisor) can follow exactly what happened during the session. Remember, if it isn't documented, it didn't happen, which can have important implications in terms of liability when others evaluate the quality and thoroughness of the services provided.

Provide the counselor's clinical impressions from the session, including the interpretation of counselor-observed behaviors and emotions (including mental status info.) and a conceptualization of the client's issues (which may align/contrast with client's view/insight).

Assessment

Provide the ICD-10 #, diagnosis and differential diagnosis with specifiers (including any provisional considerations), prognosis, evaluation of SI/HI risk, and any testing results.

Plan

Any plans or recommendations relating to the future of treatment are stated, including the next session's appointment date and time, any referrals, and homework assignments agreed to be completed. Items listed here were either already discussed in session or, if not critical, will happen at or before the very next session.

________________________ ________________________

(Clinician, Degree, Date) (Supervisor, Degree, Date)

CASE OF ABEL (ENTIRE CASE IN CHAPTER 2)

Session #6

This marks the fourth week in a row that Abel has come to therapy. He says that he is consistently taking his lunch 4 days a week and only eats out on the day he spends with some coworkers. He also has enjoyed bowling with Simon once a week in the father-son league at the local bowling alley.

At the present time, Abel wants to figure out how to confront Mary about the time she spends with Marcus. Abel thinks he has worked enough on himself and that Mary owes it to him to be honest about whether or not there is something else happening. As you reflect with him on his motivations for questioning Mary, Abel reveals that his father cheated on his mother when Abel was a teenager. Abel found out about the incident and threatened to reveal the truth to his mother. His father called him the equivalent of a "good-for-nothing, lazy ass." Unwilling for Simon to experience the same conflict, Abel says he must know the truth and whether it is time to end his marriage. You thank Abel for his honesty and the courage to be vulnerable in session. Abel agrees to do journal writing over the course of the next week to give himself time to reflect on how he wants to move forward in a way that is healthiest for himself, Mary, and Simon. He says the plan is to take time each morning before he drives his route to do the journaling.

DAP SESSION NOTE

Client Name: Abel Tesfaye
Session Date: 5/21/2024
Session Number: 6

	Type of Session:		Nature of Contact:
	Individual	X	Scheduled Appointment
	Group		Walk-in
	Couples		Emergency
	Family		

Data: Client arrived on time for scheduled appointment. He reported successfully bringing his lunch as he has planned and has engaged in activities with his son. Client appeared agitated in the session when discussing his relationship with his wife and sad when talking about his father's infidelity.

Assessment (Include *ICD-10* # diagnosis and differential diagnosis(es):

Diagnosis: F33.2 major depressive disorder, recurrent, severe without psychotic features

Differential Diagnosis: F34.1 dysthymic disorder

F43.21 adjustment disorder with depressed mood

Prognosis remains fair at this time. Client reports compliance with interventions implementation and that depressive symptoms have reduced to two negative spirals in the past week as opposed to the previously recorded four. When asked how well therapy has been working on a scale of 1–10, client responded with an 8.

Plan: Client will journal each day for the next week and will discuss themes at the next session. He will also continue a healthy lunch routine and spend time with his son in line with treatment plan goals. Clinician provided information to client about community nutritional program Healthy Bodies, Healthy Minds.

Next scheduled appointment is 5/28/2024.

Tara Pist, MEd ______________________________

Clinician Signature ______________________________

CASE OF SUSAN—SOAP NOTE (ENTIRE CASE IN CHAPTER 2)

SOAP SESSION NOTE

Client Name: Susan Woods
Session Date: July 11, 2024
Session Number: 3

	Type of Session:		Nature of Contact:
X	Individual	X	Scheduled Appointment
	Group		Walk-in
	Couples		Emergency
	Family		

Subjective: Client reported feeling increasingly anxious as a result of being a grad student and a recent move, after the death of her husband. She mentioned having trouble sleeping, racing thoughts, and stomachaches. Client indicated that she feels somewhat better when talking to friends or practicing mindfulness exercises but that this relief is temporary at best, saying, "I can't stop thinking about all the things that I don't know how to do and feel like I am not doing well in my grad program."

Objective: Client appeared visibly tense, frequently fidgeting with her hands. Her speech was rapid, and she had a furrowed brow. Client maintained good eye contact throughout the session but showed signs of agitation, such as tapping her foot.

Assessment (Include *ICD-10* # diagnosis and differential diagnosis(es):

Diagnosis: F43.23 adjustment disorder with mixed anxiety and depressed mood

Differential diagnosis: F41.1 generalized anxiety disorder

F32 major depressive disorder

Client is experiencing heightened anxiety related to studies and life transition, consistent with diagnosis of adjustment disorder with anxiety. Her reported symptoms (difficulty sleeping, racing thoughts, and stomachaches) are consistent with anxiety. Client has shown progress with coping strategies but remains significantly stressed with her studies and life transition.

Plan: Validate client's feelings about her studies and normalize her anxiety as a common reaction to significant life changes. Practice deep-breathing exercises together during session to help client manage immediate anxiety symptoms. Work on helping client to build overall resilience to life changes and stressors through ongoing therapy sessions. Explore and address any underlying issues contributing to anxiety and adjustment difficulties. Explore any new stressors or triggers that may have arisen, and adjust coping strategies accordingly.

<u>Recommended Services and Community Referrals:</u>

Support Groups: Client may benefit from joining a bereavement support group as well as a support group for graduate students experiencing stress and anxiety. Gone But Not Forgotten, (555) 243-7692
Mindfulness and Stress Reduction Programs: Client may benefit from attending local mindfulness workshops and/or yoga classes. Inner Peace Fitness, (555) 243-8322
Academic Support Services: Client may benefit from university counseling services or academic support services for academic coaching and workshops on study skills and time and stress management skills.

Gene Hudlow, MEd, LPCC ______________________________

Clinician Signature__________________________

CASE OF SUSAN—DAP NOTE (ENTIRE CASE IN CHAPTER 2)

DAP SESSION NOTE

Client Name: Susan Woods
Session Date: 6/18/2024
Session Number: 2

	Type of Session:		Nature of Contact:
X	Individual	X	Scheduled Appointment
	Group		Walk-in
	Couples		Emergency
	Family		

Data: Client reported feeling overwhelmed and anxious about her studies. She described having trouble sleeping, racing thoughts, and stomachaches. Susan mentioned feeling better when she talks about things and practices mindfulness exercises.

Assessment (Include *ICD-10* # diagnosis and differential diagnosis(es):

Diagnosis: F43.23 adjustment disorder with mixed anxiety and depressed mood

Differential Diagnosis: F41.1 generalized anxiety disorder

F32 major depressive disorder

Client is experiencing heightened anxiety related to her studies and self-expectations, consistent with her diagnosis of adjustment disorder with anxiety. Her sleep disturbances and physical symptoms (stomachaches) are indicative of her anxious state. Client has shown progress in using coping strategies, such as talking to friends and mindfulness exercises, which she reports provide temporary relief. However, her anxiety about her studies and life transition remains a significant stressor.

Plan: Validate client's feelings about study stressors and normalize her anxiety as a common reaction to life changes. Practice deep-breathing exercises together during the session to help manage immediate anxiety symptoms.

Recommended Services and Community Referrals:
Support Groups: Client may benefit from joining a bereavement support group as well as a support group for graduate students experiencing stress and anxiety. Gone But Not Forgotten, (555) 243-7692
Mindfulness and Stress Reduction Programs: Client may benefit from attending local mindfulness workshops and/or yoga classes. Inner Peace Fitness, (555) 243-8322
Academic Support Services: Client may benefit from university counseling services or academic support services for academic coaching and workshops on study skills and time and stress management skills.

Gene Hudlow, MEd, LPCC ____________________

Clinician Signature ____________________

REFERENCES

American Counseling Association. (2014). *2014 ACA code of ethics.* https://www.counseling.org/docs/

American Psychological Association (2017). *Ethical principles of psychologists and code of conduct.* https://www.apa.org/ethics/code

Baird, B. (2005). *The internship, practicum and field placement handbook: A guide for the helping professions (4th ed.).* Routledge.

Cameron, S., & turtle-song, i. (2002). Learning to write case notes using the SOAP format. *Journal of Counseling & Development, 80*, 286–292.

Dubi, M., Raggi, M., & Reynolds, J. (2012). *Distance supervision: The PIDIB model.* American Counseling Association.

Erford, B. T. (2015). *Clinical experiences in counseling.* Pearson.

Falvey, J. E., Bray, T. E., & Hebert, D. J. (2005). Case conceptualization and treatment planning: Investigation of problem-solving and clinical judgment. *Journal of Mental Health Counseling, 27*(4), 348–372.

Flückiger, C., Rubel, J., Del Re, A. C., Horvath, A. O., Wampold, B. E., Crits-Christoph, P., Atzil-Slonim, D., Compare, A., Falkenström, F., Ekeblad, A., Errázuriz, P., Fisher, H., Hoffart, A., Huppert, J. D., Kivity, Y., Kumar, M., Lutz, W., Muran, J. C., Strunk, D. R. ... Barber, J. P. (2020). The reciprocal relationship between alliance and early treatment symptoms: A two-stage individual participant data meta-analysis. *Journal of Consulting and Clinical Psychology, 88*(9), 829–843. https://doi.org/10.1037/ccp0000594

Hartsell, T. L., Jr., & Bernstein, B. E. (2008). *The portable ethicist for mental health professionals: A complete guide to responsible practice, with HIPAA update (2nd ed.).* John Wiley & Sons.

Hutchinson, M., Casper, P., Harris, J., Orcutt, J., & Trejo, M. (2008). *The clinician's guide to writing treatment plans and progress notes: For the DADS adult system of care.*

Kodweis, K., Schimmelfing, L. C., Yang, Y., & Persky, A. M. (2021). Methods for optimizing student pharmacist learning of clinical note writing. *American Journal of Pharmaceutical Education, 85*(2), 144–151.

Lambert, M. (2004). Fifty years of psychotherapy process-outcome research: Continuity and change. In M. Lambert (Ed.), *Bergin and Garfield's handbook of psychotherapy and behavior change* (5th ed.). John Wiley & Sons.

McCulloch, G. (2023). *Good practice guidelines: Writing session notes.* Psychotherapy and Counselling Federation of Australia. https://pacfa.org.au/common/Uploaded files/PCFA/Documents/Documents and Forms/Writing Session Notes.pdf

National Association of Social Workers. (2021). *Code of ethics of the National Association of Social Workers.* https://www.socialworkers.org/About/Ethics/Code-of-Ethics/Code-of-Ethics

Piazza, N. J., & Baruth, N. E. (1990). Client record guidelines. *Journal of Counseling & Development, 68*, 313–316.

Prieto, L. R., & Scheel, K. R. (2002). Using case documentation to strengthen counselor trainees' case conceptualization skills. *Journal of Counseling & Development, 80*, 11–21.

Raggi, M., Dubi, M., & Reynolds, J. (2008). The use of a pantheoretical case note format as clinical tool. *The New Jersey Journal of Professional Counseling, 60*, 5–11.

Reiter, M. D., & Sabo, K. (2023). Writing progress notes. In M. D. Reiter (Ed.), *A therapist's guide to writing in psychotherapy: Assessment, documentation, and intervention* (pp. 18–41). Routledge. https://doi.org/10.4324/9781003294702-1

Sperry, L. (2005). Case conceptualization: The missing link between theory and practice. *The Family Journal: Counseling and Therapy for Couples and Families, 13*(1), 71–76.

Standards for Privacy of Individually Identifiable Health Information, 45 C.F.R. § 160, 164 (2000).

Weed, L. L. (1968). Medical records that guide and teach. *New England Journal of Medicine, 278*(11), 593–600.

Zhang, N., & Parsons, R. D. (2016). *Field experience: Transitioning from student to professional.* Sage. https://doi.org/10.4135/9781483398709

CHAPTER 9

Discharge or Termination Summary

Melinda Mays, EdD, Gregory L. Bohner, PhD, Darlene Vaughn, PhD, Holly J. Mattingly, PhD, Mona Gallo, EdD, and Marisa L. White, PhD

INTRODUCTION

As in all stages of treatment, the end of treatment also requires documentation. The final piece of clinical documentation for a client who is ending services is typically referred to as a *discharge summary* or *termination summary*, and in this chapter, these terms will be used interchangeably. The termination summary is a comprehensive document prepared by a clinician at the conclusion of a client's mental health treatment. This summary encapsulates the key aspects of the therapeutic process and often includes a summary of the goals and progress made in treatment.

PURPOSE OF A TERMINATION SUMMARY

The termination summary is important for a variety of reasons. Primarily, the termination summary captures the course of treatment and its outcomes (Piazza & Baruth, 1990). In addition, thorough documentation is an ethical mandate. Documents like the treatment summary help to provide accountability and transparency about the counseling process, including the termination of treatment. A termination summary can also be helpful for legal protection. Should a dispute arise about treatment, the termination summary may offer critical evidence of the care provided. In fact, if a client decides to terminate treatment prematurely, proper documentation is recommended to decrease potential liability (Erford, 2015; GoodTherapy, 2019; Hodges, 2021).

The termination summary also provides closure. The termination synopsis is a formal document that indicates the conclusion of the counseling relationship. This closure can provide clients with a sense of completion, helping them to recognize and celebrate the progress they made in treatment. This closure can also help promote client autonomy and reduce unhealthy dependence on the counselor.

Termination summaries also provide an opportunity to evaluate the treatment. In addition, summarizing the treatment allows the counselor and client to reflect on the counseling process. Reflecting on the therapeutic outcomes and the client's progress contributes to the counselor's professional development. It is an opportunity to evaluate the effectiveness of the therapeutic approaches and interventions. Clients could also use the information in the summary to reflect on their goals and the treatment outcomes.

Treatment summary documentation may also be helpful in future planning. Oftentimes, termination plans include recommendations for the future. This can help the client with aftercare and foster self-efficacy. Termination summaries also provide helpful information for continuity of care. These documents help the new clinician understand the client's history and what was included in previous treatment. For example, if a client moves to a different state or changes providers for another reason, it may be helpful for the new clinician to have a summary treatment to help with the transition.

WHEN TO PRESENT TREATMENT TERMINATION

Clients leave treatment for various reasons, and clinicians need to discuss termination of services well in advance of the actual discharge (Hodges, 2021). As previously mentioned in this textbook, considering and discussing termination or discharge starts long before the client reaches this stage of treatment. In fact, effective clinicians incorporate thinking about termination into their first and concurrent meetings with the client (Erford, 2015). Counseling is intended to assist the client in developing skills and insights that will help them reach their optimal level of functioning without becoming dependent on the clinician and therapy sessions. Discussing termination throughout treatment can help ensure that the client is aware that treatment is temporary and that healthy termination of treatment is a goal.

Ideally, the client will continue in services until both the clinician and the client believe the termination of services is appropriate. However, this requires a level of commitment from the client, and some clients may not be able to reach the ideal conclusion of treatment. Research shows that of those that do return after the initial session, the median length of counseling is typically 4–6 sessions (Hatchett, 2020). Regardless of whether the client stays in counseling until goals are reached or they drop out early, it is extremely important to document the process and what happened.

ETHICAL NEED FOR DOCUMENTING A DISCHARGE OR TERMINATION SUMMARY

Although most codes of ethics for clinicians do not specifically mention the necessity of the termination summary, the *2014 ACA Code of Ethics* (American Counseling Association [ACA], 2014), *Ethical Principles of Psychologists and Code of Conduct* (American Psychological Association [APA], 2017), and the *Code of Ethics of the National Association of Social Workers* (National Association of Social Workers [NASW], 2021) all contain some statement about the necessity of developing and maintaining accurate and thorough documentation. Clinicians need to take reasonable steps and ensure the client file documentation is an accurate reflection of client progress and the services provided. Preparing a client for termination or the steps taken to ensure client welfare when they drop out early are services that need to be documented (ACA, 2014; APA, 2017; NASW, 2021).

The ideal scenario is that the client has reached the goals of the treatment plan and the clinician helps the client transition to a life without regular counseling sessions. This transition would also be documented in a well-developed termination summary. If a client "drops out" of counseling prematurely, this does not negate the need for documenting a termination summary. If a client disappears from the schedule, an ethical clinician will try to contact the client to ascertain the reason for the early termination and encourage the client to continue trying to reach their agreed-upon goals and offer alternative resources as appropriate. Most agencies will have a protocol for addressing clients who stop coming to counseling. Even in absence, these are counseling services that need to be documented.

Clinicians are charged with the responsibility for sufficient and timely creation, protection, and overall maintenance of case documentation that is reflective of client progress and services provided (ACA, 2014; APA, 2017; NASW, 2021). If amendments are made to client records and documentation, clinicians need to properly record the amendments according to agency or institutional policies (ACA, 2014).

Discharging a client from treatment is optimally done when it becomes reasonably apparent that the client no longer needs assistance, is not likely to benefit from continuing, or is being harmed by continued counseling (ACA, 2014; APA, 2017; NASW, 2021). Clinicians should not terminate services for self-gratifying pursuits (NASW, 2021). A clinician may terminate counseling if in jeopardy of harm by the client or by someone with whom the client has a relationship or when clients do not pay agreed-upon fees (ACA, 2014; APA, 2017; NASW, 2021). If there is voluntary or involuntary employment separation, the clinician is responsible for informing clients of appropriate options for the continuation of services and of the benefits and risks of the options (NASW, 2021).

Ethical clinicians take reasonable steps to avoid abandoning clients who are still in need of services, withdrawing services precipitously only under unusual circumstances. Clinicians need to minimize possible adverse effects on the client by making appropriate arrangements for continuation of services when necessary (ACA, 2014; APA, 2017; NASW, 2021). An ideal client discharge provides space for clinicians to offer pre-termination counseling and recommend other service providers when necessary, working to ensure that appropriate clinical and administrative processes are completed and open communication is maintained with all parties (ACA, 2014; APA, 2017).

Referrals are often part of a client's discharge process and can serve multiple purposes. If there is anticipated termination or a known interruption of services, the clinician should include a prompt notification to the client. The client can then choose to be transferred, referred, or pause and then continue services with the same clinician. The clinician should consider a referral to other professionals with specialized knowledge or expertise when it could benefit the client (APA, 2017; NASW, 2021). Clinicians become knowledgeable about culturally and clinically appropriate referral resources and offer referrals if they self-determine they lack the competence to be of professional assistance to clients, especially when the counselor's values are inconsistent with the client's goals or are discriminatory in nature, wherein they then discontinue the relationship (ACA, 2014). The ethical clinician needs to take appropriate steps to expedite an orderly transfer of responsibility and to disclose to those appointed by the client's consent and release of information (see Chapter 4; NASW, 2021).

After a treatment episode is completed, the ACA (2014) ethical code indicates that clinicians are responsible for storing clients' records to ensure reasonable future access and to maintain compliance with federal and state laws and statutes, and after the allotted time frame, they are to dispose of client records and other sensitive materials in a manner that protects client confidentiality. Special care is to be given to destroying client records that may be needed in a court of law, such as notation of child abuse, suicide, sexual harassment, or violence.

LEGAL NEED FOR DOCUMENTING A DISCHARGE OR TERMINATION SUMMARY

It is important to maintain accurate records for both the client's welfare and protection of the clinician (Piazza & Baruth, 1990). While the law does not specifically detail the need for a termination summary, it does emphasize the need for accurate documentation of all phases of the counseling process. In fact, record keeping is one of the top five areas for a clinician's legal liability (Piazza & Baruth, 1990).

One instance of a legal need for documentation of discharge or termination summary would be if the client would file a complaint against the clinician. A thorough termination summary would show all the actions of the clinician with supporting details. Providing a summary of a client's progress with a goal-oriented and hopeful plan for the future is helpful in the immediate provision of services and for future engagements (Erford, 2015). This is true whether the client's termination was agreed upon or a result of the client leaving services early.

Each state has specific laws and/or administrative regulations related to termination, referral, and discharge. Clinicians should seek guidance from their state regulations and/or state licensing boards to determine the regulations specified by their state government. A termination summary is an essential requirement because it depicts the services provided to the client, the rationale for discharge, referrals, and the reason services are no longer needed. If the client needs additional services, such as a higher level of care or specialized expertise to address a specific need, the clinician should provide the names of the facilities and contact information for the referral to assist the client in the continuity of services. The discharge summary should be signed and dated by the clinician and added to the client's file. Typically, this occurs within a 30-day period of the client being discharged.

INSURANCE PURPOSES IN DOCUMENTING A DISCHARGE OR TERMINATION SUMMARY

Most third-party payments come from private insurance companies and governmental programs (Erford, 2015). Third-party payers have a duty to ensure that services are delivered in an accurate and cost-effective manner. This requires the clinician's cooperation in providing documentation of exactly which services were provided and for what reasons. This documentation applies to every step in the counseling process, up to and including termination.

WHAT IS INCLUDED IN THE DISCHARGE TERMINATION AND WHY

There is no universally accepted format of what a termination summary should look like; however, as in other components of treatment documentation, there is a general consensus of what should be included. Many agencies use a template for a discharge summary, which can be helpful, but it is important that the template be modified as needed to specifically reflect the client's situation, including multicultural concerns (TheraPlatform, n.d.). The contents of a termination summary are a synopsis of the assessment, the client's identified problems initial diagnosis(es), differential diagnosis(es), diagnosis at discharge, the presenting problems, the goals and outcomes of treatment, final outcomes for each identified problem, an evaluation of their current functioning, the reason for discharge or termination, and referrals (Piazza & Baruth, 1990; TheraPlatform, n.d.). There may be differences in the labels used, but the sections are usually very similar across discharge summary documents. Clinicians who include information for each of these topics would yield a well-developed termination summary.

Ideally, the client would be involved in the creation of the termination summary. Including the client may help to ensure that they understand the recommendations and may increase the likelihood of follow-through (TheraPlatform, n.d.). It is important that the language in the termination documents, as in other documents in the case file, be clear and concise. This is even more true when termination is the client's choice. The clinician should always report facts in language that does not blame the client.

Case Note

The clinician will provide a clear report of how and when the case termination was handled, usually in a final session note. The case note for the session needs to include which preparation strategies were used. Strategies typically used include an iteration of the therapeutic process, processing of the client's feelings about ending the treatment relationships, reflection on the client's growth and plans for continued growth, and when it may be appropriate to return to therapy (GoodTherapy, 2019).

Some agencies may use a mental health maintenance plan or similar document to clarify for the client how to proceed with maintaining their mental health. This would remind the clients of triggers that have been identified and strategies for managing them with skills learned in therapy, such as coping skills, self-care, and social support. It would also include warning signs to help the client identify that the presenting problem might be returning so they will know when to employ coping strategies or possibly return to counseling (GoodTherapy, 2019). If this is used, it should also become part of the termination summary

Reason for Discharge or Termination

As mentioned before, discharge or termination is ideally reached when the client has met their therapeutic goals (Barnett & Coffman, 2015). Regardless of whether that is the case or not, the client's termination summary needs to clearly define the reason for discharge or termination in factual, nonjudgmental language (GoodTherapy, 2019). If termination is occurring because the client has reached their goals, then inclusion of evidence to that effect would be important. If termination is occurring for other reasons, such as counseling no longer being beneficial, lack of client engagement, no-shows, lack of payment, and so on, then that should be described in factual terms.

Initial Diagnosis(es), Differential Diagnosis(es) and Diagnosis at Discharge

Much of the treatment process is based on the client's diagnosis. Since the discharge summary includes the beginning, the middle, and the end of the client's counseling process, inclusion of the initial diagnosis is important. Providing a differential diagnosis supports the initial diagnosis as the most accurate description of the client, which was evidenced by the consideration and rejection of similar diagnoses. Often, as the clinician comes to know the client or as the client progresses, the clinician may determine that the initial diagnosis is no longer accurate. Providing a diagnosis at discharge ensures that any future clinician will get the most accurate description of the client.

Presenting Problems

Since the termination summary describes the whole counseling process, clinicians are guided to document the client's presenting problem(s) that first brought the client into services, which usually determine the basis for the goals in the client's treatment plan. This information is often demonstrative of outcome measures for client growth, stagnation, or recidivist behaviors.

Goals of Treatment

As previously determined, an integral component of the counseling process is the establishment of goals. These goals direct treatment and provide a clear vision for both the client and the clinician. Perhaps the most important purpose, however, is to provide specific criteria for the termination of the counseling services. The fundamental goal of counseling is to assist the client in returning to a satisfactory, if not optimal, state of functioning without dependence on the clinician. The client's goals tailor this to specific criteria that are unique to the client's situation. Including the goals and the status of these goals in the discharge summary forms the basis for showing that termination is appropriate.

Referrals

Clinicians are responsible for providing the client with notice of termination as well as the opportunity to procure the services of another health professional (Barnett & Coffman, 2015). Clients may be concerned about having support once therapy has ended (GoodTherapy, 2019). A client may resist termination because they have made a connection with the clinician, may have only a few close relationships, or fear their ability to sustain their recovery regimen (Hodges, 2021). Offering referral sources can help the client feel supported once therapy has ended. If a direct referral to an adjunct provider is supplied to the client, then the name and contact information of the referral needs to be documented (Cameron & turtle-song, 2002). Documenting at least three referral sources for current needs identified through client collaboration is an important part of the termination summary.

TERMINATION LETTER

A common practice in clinical work is to send a termination letter to clients upon the close of the counseling relationship. If a termination letter has been sent to the client, it is imperative for the clinician to make a notation of this as part of the termination summary. Sending a termination letter is a courtesy, not necessarily a part of the documentation of termination. Although sending a letter is often an agency decision, in some situations a termination letter is recommended.

One instance where a termination letter would be important is when a discharge occurs because of client behavior, such as repeated no-shows, when the client is considered a threat to the clinician or someone close to the clinician, or when someone repeatedly threatens legal action (GoodTherapy, 2019). Another situation is when the clinician determines that termination would be in the client's best interest so they can pursue a more appropriate counseling provider. A final recommendation for sending a termination letter is that it demonstrates the clinician attempt to communicate a very clear explanation of the reason for the client's counseling termination (GoodTherapy, 2019).

CONCLUSION

It may be tempting, once therapy has ended, to feel that the duty for documentation has been fulfilled; however, the termination or discharge summary is just as important as any other piece of clinical documentation. The discharge summary provides a clear description of what occurred during the counseling process and the reasons for termination, as well as steps for self-maintenance and after-care referrals.

A concise, detailed termination or discharge summary presents multiple benefits. The benefits for the client are that there is a clear record available for continuity of care if the client returns to therapy. In the case of agreed-upon termination, the discharge summary serves as a reminder to the client of what they have accomplished and ways they can move forward in maintaining their own mental health.

A benefit for the clinician is the summary of actions taken by the clinician that includes the clinical rationale. This can be helpful if the client returns for more therapy or if the client should make a complaint against the clinician. Not only does a termination summary provide a memory aid for the clinician but it may also be submitted as evidence if the need arises, which makes this piece of the documentation just as important as the documentation of assessment, treatment planning, and ongoing services.

CASE OF ABEL (ENTIRE CASE IN CHAPTER 2)

Session #10

Abel has missed 3 out of the last 4 weeks of sessions. He calls the day before to reschedule for the next week at the same time. At the beginning of the current session, you reiterate the importance of working consistently in order to achieve Abel's goals of increasing his mental wellbeing and strengthening the relationship with his family. As a way of bolstering his work so far, you reflect on the progress he has made in exercising consistently, eating a healthier diet, and spending time with Simon. You ask whether the day and time are still the best fit for Abel's schedule. As you are talking, Abel appears to become more agitated. When you ask what his current thoughts are, Abel says therapy is obviously a waste of time. Angrily, he says, "All of the things you told me to do haven't changed anything!" He reveals that Mary still cheated on him with Marcus. It is only 15 minutes into the session, but Abel storms out. You call him later that day to discuss rescheduling so he can talk further about how he wants to move forward, but he does not return any of your phone calls or emails over the course of the next week. You complete his termination letter and add it to his client file. Finally, you schedule a reminder to call one more time a week later to attempt to reestablish a connection and provide an opportunity for further sessions or referrals to other therapists.

FINAL SESSION/TERMINATION EVENT SUMMARY

Client Name: Abel Tesfaye
Date: 07/30/24
Session: 10

Data: Client arrived on time for scheduled appointment. Clinician discussed whether to change the scheduled time, as client had rescheduled 3 out of the past 4 weeks. As the session progressed, client became visibly frustrated and disengaged. Clinician reflected on the nonverbal communication, and client expressed displeasure at the progress of therapy regarding his marriage and exited the session before the end of the session. Client has not responded to clinician's attempts to communicate by phone and email.

Assessment (Include *ICD-10* # diagnosis and differential diagnosis(es):

Diagnosis: F33.2 major depressive disorder, recurrent, severe without psychotic features

Differential Diagnosis: F34.1 dysthymic disorder

F43.21 adjustment disorder with depressed mood

Prognosis remains fair at this time. Client met the first goal of the treatment plan, but consistent implementation of interventions is needed for continued decrease of symptoms.

Plan: Clinician will mail discharge summary to client with referral sources and invitation to reengage in services in the future. File will be closed at this time.

Main reason for termination of services:

	The planned treatment was completed.
X	The client refused to receive or participate in services.
	There was little or no progress in treatment.
	This is a planned extended pause in treatment.
	The client was referred for services elsewhere. The client was referred to:
	Other:

Source of termination decision:

X	Client initiated.		Clinician initiated.
	Mutual decision.		Other:

Presenting Problem(s):

Client is returning home after hospitalization from suicidal ideation and wants to address his depressive symptoms. In addition, he wants to improve the relationship with his spouse so that it becomes "more bearable."

Goal(s) of Therapy:

Client will:

1. Learn three coping strategies to mitigate depressive symptomology by 50% occurrences in a month—Goal met 5/28/2024.
2. Increase positive communication patterns with spouse to three positive conversations a week—Goal not met and discontinued by client on 7/30/2024.

Referrals:

Ms. Pist

Moving Past Affairs Support Group: (555) 217-6923

Western Samaritan Hospital: (555) 216-7373

No signature obtained as client left session and will not respond to messages

Client Signature

CASE OF SUSAN (ENTIRE CASE IN CHAPTER 2)

FINAL SESSION/TERMINATION EVENT SUMMARY

Client Name: Susan Woods
Date: 11/1/2024
Session: 12

Subjective: Client reported feeling significantly better and more in control of her anxiety and grief. Client indicated that while initially things were tough, she has found increasing stability through regular practice of coping strategies discussed and reviewed in therapy. Client feels increasingly confident in her ability to manage her academic stress and has developed a supportive routine that includes mindfulness exercises and social interactions.

Objective: Client appeared calm and composed during the termination session. Client maintained good eye contact and showed no sign of agitation. Client's speech was steady and clear, and she displayed a relaxed posture, with no fidgeting or signs of distress observed.

Assessment (Include *ICD-10* # diagnosis and differential diagnosis(es):

Diagnosis: F43.23 adjustment disorder with mixed anxiety and depressed mood

Differential Diagnosis: F41.1 generalized anxiety disorder

F32 major depressive disorder

Client has made significant progress in reducing symptoms of anxiety and grief. Client has developed effective coping strategies for managing her grief and academic stress and has learned techniques for improving her emotional regulation. The goals of therapy have been met, and client feels confident in her ability to manage ongoing challenges independently.

Plan: Encourage client to continue utilizing community resources to maintain her progress and build a robust support network. Follow up with client in a month to check on adjustment and make any new necessary recommendations and referrals.

Main reason for termination of services:

X	The planned treatment was completed.
	The client refused to receive or participate in services.
	There was little or no progress in treatment.
	This is a planned extended pause in treatment.
	The client was referred for services elsewhere. The client was referred to:
	Other:

Source of termination decision:

	Client initiated.		Therapist initiated.
X	Mutual decision.		Other:

Presenting Problem(s):

Client is experiencing anxiety and stress related to recent changes and life stressors. She has recently experienced the loss of spouse, a significant move, new home, returned to being a full-time student after not expecting to ever return to school, change in income, change in life direction.

Goal(s) of Therapy:

Client will:

1. Reduce symptoms of severe anxiety and grief.
2. Develop coping strategies for grief.
3. Manage academic stress.
4. Learn to enhance emotional regulation.

Referrals:

Gone But Not Forgotten: (555) 243-7692

Inner Peace Fitness: (555) 243-8322

Grand Towers College Academic Center: (555) 839-4242

Susan Woods ______________________________

Client Signature

REFERENCES

American Counseling Association. (2014). *2014 ACA code of ethics.* https://www.counseling.org/docs/

American Psychological Association. (2017). *Ethical principles of psychologists and code of conduct.* https://www.apa.org/ethics/code

Barnett, J. E., & Coffman, C. (2015, June). *Termination and abandonment: A proactive approach to ethical practice.* Society for the Advancement of Psychotherapy. https://societyforpsychotherapy.org/termination-and-abandonment-a-proactive-approach-to-ethical-practice/

Cameron, S., & turtle-song, i. (2002). Learning to write case notes using the SOAP format. *Journal of Counseling & Development, 80,* 286–292.

Erford, B. (2015). *Clinical experiences in counseling.* Pearson.

GoodTherapy. (2019, August 7). *How to navigate the termination of therapy with a client.* https://www.goodtherapy.org/for-professionals/business-management/private-practices/article/how-to-navigate-the-termination-of-therapy-with-a-client

Hatchett, G. T. (2020). Anticipating and planning for the duration of counseling. *Journal of Mental Health Counseling, 42,* 1–14.

Hodges, S. (2021). *The counseling practicum and internship manual: A resource for counseling graduate students* (3rd ed.). Springer.

National Association of Social Work. (2021). *Code of ethics of the National Association of Social Workers.* https://www.socialworkers.org/About/Ethics/Code-of-Ethics/Code-of-Ethics

Piazza, N. J., & Baruth, N. E. (1990). In the field: Client record guidelines. *Journal of Counseling & Development, 68,* 313–316.

TheraPlatform. (n.d.). *Therapy discharge plan.* Retrieved April 28, 2024, from https://www.theraplatform.com/blog/1011/therapy-discharge-plan

CHAPTER 10

Ethical Issues and Crisis Documentation

Marisa L. White, PhD, Mona Gallo, EdD, Darlene Vaughn, PhD, Gregory L. Bohner, PhD, and Holly J. Mattingly, PhD

INTRODUCTION

Documentation could be divided into two categories: primary and secondary. *Primary documentation* consists of the documents that are in all client's records, including the informed consent, release of information, case notes, a treatment plan, and termination summary. *Secondary documents* are records that occur for some clients or specific situations. For example, some client files may have a referral form because the client qualifies for case management services. Other instances would be assessment and testing results, or some clients may require additional documentation due to a crisis or ethical concerns. This chapter details documenting ethical issues and crisis situations.

DOCUMENTING ETHICAL ISSUES

Ethical guidelines in treatment are vitally important considerations for clinicians. *Ethics* refers to the moral principles that guide a counselor's behavior and decision-making, while *laws* are the legal regulations that govern the practice of therapy. Ethical guidelines, such as those outlined by the American Counseling Association (ACA, 2014), the National Association of Social Workers (NASW, 2021), and the American Psychological Association (APA, 2017), provide clinicians with standards for professional conduct, confidentiality, boundaries, and client welfare. These guidelines are designed to promote the well-being of clients and ensure clinicians act in an ethical manner.

On the other hand, therapy-related laws are legal regulations that govern the practice of counseling and are enforced by state licensing boards and professional organizations. These laws address issues such as licensure requirements, scope of practice, informed consent, and mandatory reporting of child abuse and harm to self or others. It is important for clinicians to be aware of both ethical guidelines and legal regulations to provide competent and ethically sound care to clients. Violating ethical guidelines or laws can result in disciplinary action, loss of licensure, or legal consequences, or a combination thereof.

Clinicians may find documenting ethical concerns difficult for multiple reasons. First, ethical concerns can ignite different emotions in clinicians, and documenting such occurrences may provoke anxiety. Second, these documents could be reviewed to assess the ethical behavior of the clinician, which could possibly impact the clinician's job, licensure status, or legal findings (i.e., malpractice, negligence). Third, there is no specific form or format that is used to document ethical concerns, as they are typically specific to the agency or clinician. Finally, there is no standard location where this documentation is kept, as document maintenance rests on the situation, agency, and clinician.

When documenting ethical concerns, it is important to document factual, objective, and verifiable information rather than personal opinions and feelings. It is also important to remember that all documents about ethical concerns, even personal records, may be viewed by people or entities outside of the client. These can include but may not be limited to lawyers, licensure boards, courts, or consultants. For these reasons, all documentation should be written in a professional manner. This is important to reiterate here because some ethical documentation may be kept in the client file, while other documents may be in a supervision note or personal note. Regardless of the location of the documentation, professionalism in the content is critical.

Despite there being no industry format required to document ethical concerns, the *2014 ACA Codes of Ethics* (ACA, 2014), the *National Association of Social Work Code of Ethics* (NASW, 2021), and the *Ethical Principles of Psychologists and Code of Conduct* (APA, 2017) indicate what information must be documented concerning ethical situations. For example, if a clinician decides to extend ethical boundaries (e.g., attend a client's graduation ceremony or funeral), the clinician would address such precautions through informed consent, consultation, and supervision. The entire decision-making process should be documented (ACA, 2014). Curiously, both the NASW (2021) and the APA (2017) are silent on the documentation of any boundary extensions but do indicate when to document ethical concerns regarding informed consent and disclosures. Even though the *ACA's* (2014) ethical code guides the clinician's choices, there is no distinction about how or where to document ethical concerns or how these documents are to be retained. This leaves the burden of decision-making surrounding the documentation to the agency or individual counselor.

ETHICAL DECISION-MAKING PROCESS

When an ethical concern or dilemma arises, only the counseling profession recommends a clinician use an ethical decision-making model to navigate the ethical matter (ACA, 2014; American Mental Health Counselors Association [AMHCA], 2020). In the code of ethics for the NASW (2021) and the APA (2017), there are no direct references to the use of a decision-making model to navigate or plot a course of action in response to an ethical concern.

Both the AMHCA (2020) and the ACA (2014) suggest that clinicians document how they progress through an ethical decision-making model when they experience an ethical concern. While the AMHCA (2020) recommends the use of their six-step model of ethical decision-making, the ACA (2014) notes only that counselors use an ethical decision-making model.

There are many ethical decision-making models that clinicians could use when navigating ethical decisions. Clinicians, in most instances, may choose and use the ethical decision-making model of their choice. It is best practice to review ethical decision-making models *before* the need to use one arises. Choosing the "best" model is a matter of professional opinion, but clinicians can look to many organizations, research, or literature to choose the ethical decision-making model that may best fit their professional situation.

Cottone and Claus (2000) summarize nine practice-based ethical decision-making models. The ACA (2014), as cited by Ling and Hauck (2017), endorses the use of the model set forth by Forester-Miller and Davis (2016) in *Practitioner's Guide to Ethical Decision Making* because this model can be used by novice and expert clinicians alike, as well as with diverse ethical concerns. Some ethical decision-making models specifically denote a step dedicated to documentation and some do not, but it is best practice and ethically sound to document all steps of the decision-making process.

ETHICAL DECISION-MAKING MODEL APPLICATION

One way to document an ethical dilemma would be to record which ethical decision-making model the clinician chose and the reasons the clinician chose that specific model. For example, a record of ethical decision-making process may read as follows: "The clinician used the model put forth in the *Practitioner's Guide to Ethical Decision Making*. This ethical decision-making model was chosen because it is supported by the ACA and considers multiple perspectives, which is important when working through ethical issues in a culturally sensitive manner."

Following best practice, the clinician would document what they did in each step. Below is an abridged example to help illustrate how a clinician might document progression through Forester-Miller and Davis's (2016) *ethical decision-making* model.

Step 1. Identify the Problem

Identify the dilemma and why it is a dilemma:
The concern: I discovered that my paramour is related to my client.
Situation: I have been dating my paramour for 8 months and recently (insert date) found out that he is related to my client. Specifically, I attended a family Christmas party with my paramour and discovered that his aunt (mother's sister) is my client. I was introduced to the client/aunt and acted like I did not know the client/aunt. At the Christmas party, I did not disclose that she was my client and I attempted to stay away from the client/aunt. On the next business day, after the party (insert date), I called the client to discuss the situation. The client has not returned the call and missed her next appointment. It should be noted that missing appointments is not uncommon for this client.

Step 2. Apply the Relevant Code of Ethics

Use the ethical code congruent with your profession. For this example, the author will use the *2014 ACA Code of Ethics* (ACA, 2014):

- A.4.a. Avoiding Harm
- A.5.a. Sexual and/or Romantic Relationships Prohibited (prohibiting sexual relationships with a client's relative)
- B.1.c. Respect for Confidentiality
- B.1.d. Explanation of Limitations
- I.1.a. Knowledge (of standards)
- I.1.b. Ethical Decision Making
- I.2.c. Consultation

Step 3. Determine the Nature and Dimension of the Dilemma

Think ahead: Identify stakeholders and how the decisions can impact each.

- Stakeholders impacted: client, counselor, partner, agency, new clinician
- Possible outcomes of each potential decision (positive [P] and negative [N]):

	REFER THE CLIENT	STOP DATING THE PARTNER	STOP ATTENDING FAMILY FUNCTIONS
CLIENT	P: The client could agree and get along well with the next counselor. N: The client could feel abandoned or punished. N: The client may not have a connection to the next counselor.	P: Not impact the client at all N: Feeling guilty for breaking up the family member's relationship	P: Not impact the client at all N: Feeling guilty due to the family member
COUNSELOR	Fill in appropriate information when retrieved or as needed.	P: Keeping the client on the load N: Resentment toward the client for breaking up the relationship	Fill in appropriate information when retrieved or as needed.
PARTNER	Fill in appropriate information when retrieved or as needed.	Fill in appropriate information when retrieved or as needed.	Fill in appropriate information when retrieved or as needed.
AGENCY	N: Possible loss of a client/income	Fill in appropriate information when retrieved or as needed.	Fill in appropriate information when retrieved or as needed.

WITH WHOM ONE CONSULTED	DATE AND TIME OF CONSULTATION	TYPE OF CONSULTATION	INFORMATION GAINED
LAWYER: SASHA JONES	March 2, 20XX via email to schedule an apt.	Legal	No laws were breached at this time.
SUPERVISOR: KALLIE GREEN	March 4, 20XX; 1:00p.m.–2:00p.m. Face-to-face meeting March 5, 20XX; 10:00a.m.–10:30a.m. Virtual meeting	Clinical	Consult with the client about how they would like to proceed. Ensure confidentiality of all clients by not discussing client details outside of the office.
SUPERVISOR KALLIE GREEN	(Date & Time Frame)	Ethical	Specific ethical codes were identified (as mentioned above). Options were identified. Consequences were identified.

ACA ETHICS COMMITTEE: MARISSA W.	(Date & Time Frame)		
OHIO COUNSELING ASSOCIATION ETHICS CHAIR: JAKE JOHNSON	(Date & Time Frame)		
INSURANCE CO: HPSO	(Date) via email	Risk management	See the additional risk management document attached to the file.

Step 4. Generate Possible Course of Action

Include information about the consultation. Include information about literature, regulations, laws, and how they support or discourage actions. Possible solutions:

1. Break up with my partner.
2. Transfer or refer the client to another clinician.
3. Stop attending family functions.

Step 5. Consider Potential Consequences for All Options, then Determine a Course of Action

Calculate risk, and include information about how you consider the risk for each possible decision. Select and document the selected action. Rank decisions and indicate which decision is most ethical and defensible and aligns with best practices.

Step 6. Evaluate the Selected Course of Action

Document the steps taken to ensure autonomy, justice, beneficence, nonmaleficence, and/or fidelity. If the course of action chosen creates a new ethical dilemma, return to previous steps to generate an alternate solution.

Step 7. Implement Course of Action

After implementing the best course of action from the previous six steps, follow up on the situation to assess whether the chosen actions had the anticipated effect and consequences.

The above example is a sample of how an ethical decision-making process could be implemented (step by step). This information may or may not be kept in a client's file. If the information documented does not include direct client information or the consideration of the client in the ethical decision-making process, then the supervisor may require it for their documentation, or it should be saved by the counselor in their personal notes.

In the case of the above example, this information would be included in the client chart if the clinician included the client in the decision-making process, such as the clinician speaking with the client to discuss boundaries or confidentiality. The clinician would document the above information, including the client contact on the above contact log, and place the detailed decision-making process in the client's chart in the form of a case note.

Remember, if client information is included in the document, the information should be kept confidential and according to legal and ethical standards. It is also important to keep in mind that if an ethical issue does progress to a complaint or legal action, this information could be required by a licensure board or subpoenaed by the court. This is just another reason why all documentation should be written professionally and accurately and documented at the time of the occurrence.

Choosing, using, and documenting an ethical decision-making model is a portion of risk management and may reduce ethical and legal liability. It is best practice for clinicians to have an identified ethical decision-making model available prior to needing one, as well as to understand the reasons they chose the model. Should an ethical concern arise, it is best practice for clinicians to document the use of the ethical decision-making model to process ethical concerns. Ethical concerns may be documented in the client file, only when relevant, and always kept by the clinician in their personal notes.

DOCUMENTING CRISIS SITUATIONS

Most clinicians are trained to help clients cope with crises. Clients may experience various crisis situations, including environmental (e.g., natural disaster), developmental (e.g., birth of a child, retirement), situational (e.g., car accident, house fire, domestic violence), existential (e.g., life transitions like divorce, grief, and loss), and systemic (e.g., discrimination) crises. Generally, these crises are discussed in session and documented in the case note. Because no additional documentation is needed to address these types of crises (unless it is mentioned as a referral), it does not diminish the seriousness of these crises experienced by clients.

Certain crisis situations, such as a client expressing homicidal or suicidal ideation, may warrant specific documentation. This type of documentation may provide steps to help the clinician reduce the risk to the client and to themselves, as well as limit exposure to legal and ethical liability through thorough and accurate crisis documentation.

Crisis situations may be documented in a variety of ways. Agencies often have specific crisis documents that they require the clinician to utilize to protect the client and the liability of the agency. Many agencies have specific forms to help the clinician document client suicidality, homicidal ideation, death, medical emergencies, or reported abuse. Outside of any required agency forms, clinicians working for an agency or independently may choose to keep additional documentation about the crisis to limit personal and professional liability. Whether documented in the client file or in the clinician's personal file, all crisis documentation should be clear, concise, timely, and objective.

Client crises are likely to be documented in several ways. If the client enters treatment as the result of the crisis or has a history of crises like suicide attempts, that information should be documented in the intake and assessment paperwork and placed in the client's file along with any obtained documentation from current or previous providers (e.g., hospital discharge documentation, psychiatrist, crisis stabilization). If the crisis is newer and the client broaches this subject during a session, the information will be documented in the case note. In addition to noting the crisis information in other documentation (intake, assessment, case notes), specific documents may be required based on the crisis.

The Substance Abuse and Mental Health Services Administration (SAMHSA, 2020) provides national guidelines for behavioral health crisis care. They note three core elements for a crisis system within a community are (1) a regional crisis call center, (2) a mobile crisis response team, and (3) crisis-receiving and stabilization facilities. SAMHSA stated there are few communities that have these core elements in place and still fewer that are effectively meeting the best practice guidelines.

DOCUMENTATION ABOUT SUICIDAL IDEATION, PLANS, AND ATTEMPTS

Documentation about suicidal ideation, plans, or attempts could encompass many different forms. Clinicians will likely have a document containing a summary of the crisis. This document will include details of the event. In addition to a summary of the crisis, a risk form, an assessment form, a safety plan, and follow-up documents may also be included as a part of the crisis documentation. Typically, the initial form or summary would include information about the suicidal ideation, plan, or attempts (IPA). Included in this document would be the date, time, precipitating events, history of suicidal IPA, as well as the frequency, intensity, and duration. If a client indicates that they have a plan, details about that plan must be obtained including when, where, how, access to means, and preparations being made by the client.

Many agencies and clinicians will have supplemental documents related to suicidal IPA. These documents have been known to include risk factors (e.g., hopelessness, isolation, job loss/financial problems, lack of social support, impulsivity, substance use, family members who died by suicide, etc.) and protective factors (e.g., reasons for living, positive support system, spirituality, positive coping skills, connection to others, etc.). This information may be obtained through a formal assessment or a checklist developed by the agency/clinician. Specific suicide assessments may include the Beck Scale for Suicidal Ideation, the Patient Health Questionnaire, and/or the Columbia Suicide Rating Scale. These assessments or the data from them are often kept in the client's file because they can provide information about symptoms, support a diagnosis, and indicate the severity of risk.

If a client indicates suicidal ideation or a loose plan, the clinician will likely develop a documented safety plan with and for the client. However, if the client indicates a specific plan or attempt or if the clinician believes that the client is a danger to themselves, they will likely refer them to a crisis agency or the hospital for additional assessment and hospitalization. No matter the level of crisis, the clinician needs to retain the relevant information in the client's file (i.e., assessments, safety plan, referrals, release of information for client supports, change in treatment plan).

If the client has thoughts of suicide but does not qualify for hospitalization, the clinician will likely create a safety plan with and for the client and increase clinical contact (e.g., phone check-ins, increase frequency of sessions). It is best practice for the client to develop the safety plan with the guidance of the clinician. This type of documentation may take different shapes but ultimately can help the client by including identify warning signs (triggers), internal coping strategies, people and social strategies to provide a distraction, an identified support system with contact details, professional agencies to contact, and ways to make the environment safe (Stanley & Brown, 2021).

Warning signs a clinician and client need to look for may include feeling isolated, depressed, anxious, or impulsive. They could also include active addiction or an isolated case of being under the influence of alcohol or drugs, the anniversary of a loss, feeling like a burden to others, experiencing unbearable emotional or physical pain, feeling guilt or shame, and so on. Behaviors could be another indicator or warning sign, including researching ways to die, saying goodbye to loved ones, taking dangerous risks, and giving away items.

Internal coping strategies a client and clinician should consider include positive thinking, reminding self of reasons to live, positive affirmations and self-talk, prayer, deep breathing, positive visualization, and meditation. External coping strategies include keeping busy, being social, spending time in nature, reading an uplifting book, exercising, acquiring adequate sleep, eating healthy, and so on. Helping the client identify a support network may require additional attention and consideration of cultural norms. The client should be reminded to choose people who are available, behave safely, and are able to provide support. Not all acquaintances, friends, and family members offer positive and stress-free support. In addition, it may not be culturally appropriate for some clients to discuss suicide with specific individuals. Should a client have difficulty identifying a strong outside support system, then identifying agency support will be important (e.g., counselor, case manager, crisis support line, a local crisis center, etc.). Lastly, do not forget the need to ensure environmental safety as part of the client's safety plan. This may include relocating firearms to a different location (family member's house) or giving the key of the gun safe to a family member. It could also include removing access to ropes, knives, large quantities of medication, and alcohol and drugs. This step may be better achieved with the assistance of a person from the client's support network.

Developing the safety plan can help the client increase awareness of their individualized risks and triggers. Ideally, this awareness will prompt quick action through the implementation of coping strategies. Consequently, early identification and action may hopefully reduce the thoughts and prevent the progression of suicidal thoughts in becoming a plan and action.

When documenting suicidality, it is important that the clinician is intentional with the terminology used. Clinicians should avoid ambiguous and subjective terminology, such as "self-harm" and "suicidal gestures." Instead of using phrases like "The client made a cry for help," it would be more accurate to note that the client indicated that they attempted to die by the method of suicide and indicate the date and time. The clinician might write, "The client reported, 'I took 8 Benadryl pills with the hopes of not waking up.'" Instead of noting that the client talked about hurting themselves, the clinician could document that the client stated, "I have thoughts of hurting myself. I think about who would care if I died and if anyone would attend my funeral. I would never do it but when I drink too much I sometimes think about death." Note that the second part of the examples provided more detail about the crisis and eliminated ambiguous terminology.

DOCUMENTATION ABOUT HOMICIDAL IDEATION, PLAN, AND ATTEMPTS

Much like suicidal ideation, plans, and actions, homicidal IPA must also be documented. Documentation about the thoughts or desires to hurt another person may look like that for suicidal IPA. Clinicians will likely have a document containing a summary of the homicidal IPA. In addition to a summary, a risk form, an assessment form, a safety plan, and follow-up documents may also be included as crisis documentation. It is important to include the details reported by the client, including the date, time, precipitating events, and history of homicidal IPA. It is imperative to also document the client's reported frequency, intensity, and duration of homicidal IPA. If a client indicates that they have a plan, details about that plan must be obtained, including when, where, how, access to means, and preparations being made by the client. In cases of homicidal IPA, the information the client reports is important because the clinician is often bound by duty to warn/duty to protect laws (often referred to as *Tarasoff laws*). Duty to warn laws, guidelines, and expectations may differ by state, but most states mandate clinicians to report a client to law enforcement if they make a credible threat to an identifiable witness. Other states have a broader duty to protect the general public, such as a case in Delaware that even expanded the scope of a clinician's responsibility to protect unidentified victims from intentional and unintentional harm (Knoll, 2019). It is imperative that clinicians know their specific state laws and take steps to protect people from harm.

When a client expresses homicidal IPA, the clinician should assess the risk and take steps to protect the identified victim and, as indicated above, sometimes the general public. Assessment of the homicidal risk should include gathering information about any ideation, plans, access to means, past experiences, future expectations, and protective factors. If the client has access to means and/or a plan to hurt identified people/persons, the clinician will likely take steps to hospitalize the client, notify the police about the crisis, notify the identified victim of the intended threat, and increase the frequency of clinical treatment after hospitalization (Knoll, 2019). These steps will require additional documentation. If the client is hospitalized—referred to a *crisis assessment team* or *hospital for assessment*—that information would likely be documented in a case note or in an additional document summarizing the crisis. This document would state who was contacted, why they were contacted (justification for breaking confidentiality), and explicitly note what information was shared. When informing the police and the potential victim/victims, the clinician should document who was contacted (name, position, contact information), why they were contacted (justification for breaking confidentiality), when they were contacted (date and time), and explicitly document what information was shared.

When a client discusses homicidal ideation loosely or without a plan or intent and the clinician deems that no one is in imminent danger, it is recommended the clinician create a safety plan with and for the client. The safety plan in a homicidal crisis is similar to the aforementioned suicide safety plan. The details of the safety plan should be specific to the situation and level of risk. The information recorded will likely include the warning signs (triggers), internal coping strategies, people and social strategies to provide a distraction, an identified support system with contact details, professional agencies to contact, and ways to make the environment safe (Stanley & Brown, 2021).

DOCUMENTATION ABOUT REPORTED ABUSE OR NEGLECT

When a clinician suspects abuse or neglect of a child, elder, or incapacitated individual, it is important that they collect any relevant information related to the suspected abuse or neglect. Clinicians should exercise caution when collecting such data because oftentimes the report of abuse/neglect and the time following the report can feel traumatic for the client or reporting individual. The initial fact-gathering session is often referred to as a *minimal facts interview*. The basic information should include who (is harmed and doing the harm), what happened (act or what occurred, how long, how often), where (locations of the act(s)), and when (dates, times). Also, how information is gathered is just as important as the information being obtained. The clinician must refrain from using leading or coercive questions, avoid making assumptions, and limit visualization (of abused body marks). It is imperative clinicians remain neutral and provide reassurance to the client or reporting individual.

When abuse of a child, elder, or incapacitated individual is suspected or reported, additional documentation is warranted. This information may appear in multiple locations, including the client's case note or a document developed specifically for reporting abuse and neglect to authorities. When documenting abuse or neglect, information should be fact-based. Document what the client or reporting individual stated, and use their exact words and phrases about the situation. Clinicians may also include observations and a subjective report, but indicate those clearly in the documentation with phrases such as "The clinician observed. ..."

In addition to documenting the reported details about the reported abuse or neglect, the clinicians will also document the date, time, and location of the report (phone, office, online). It is also best practice for the clinician to document if they consulted with a supervisor, other colleagues, or officials about the event and with whom they reported the information (e.g., supervisor or colleague's name, police, Adult Protective Services, Department of Child Services, etc.). When documenting who was consulted, include the individual's name, identification number, and case number, should these details apply to the situation. Lastly, clinicians will want to provide a detailed account of what information was shared with the contact person/agency and when it was shared (date and time).

CONCLUSION

It is important to reiterate that all documentation could be viewed by others, and as a result, it should be written accurately and with professionalism. In the case of crisis documentation, it is important to note that this type of documentation will more than likely be viewed by other professionals and/or agencies. Crisis documentation should be thorough and timely, as well as be informed by procedures, policies, laws, and the relevant code of ethics.

CASE OF ABEL (ENTIRE CASE IN CHAPTER 2)

Session #11

It has been 3 months since you have heard from Abel. He arrives at your office one morning at opening, full of desperation, and says he needs to see you right away. You have an open appointment and ask Abel to give you 5 minutes to prepare your office. He sits in the waiting room, continuously wringing his hands and rubbing them on his pant legs. He is wearing sweatpants and a baggy T-shirt that is too large.

When Abel enters the office, he starts talking before you can completely close the door. He starts by apologizing for the way he left your office the last time and says he was "just so upset about everything." He relays to you that he recently moved out of his house and has begun divorce proceedings with Mary. As he was cleaning out some of his belongings this morning, he noticed a book under the dining room table. When he opened it up, he realized he was reading his son's journal. It fell to the last page where it was written, "I wish Dad would just man up and do what it takes to win Mom back. But he never finishes anything he starts, so I don't think that will happen." Abel tells you this has sent him into a spiral and he cannot stop thinking about killing himself. "If my own son cannot see me as a man, perhaps I should just get out of the way and let Marcus raise him. My dad was right all along; I'm just a waste of space."

As you discuss the situation further with Abel, he shares that he was about to go back to his new apartment and get the gun that he owns to shoot himself. He knows a field not far from his work where no one goes to and it wouldn't make a fuss. But before reaching the apartment, he started worrying about whether or not he should go through with it and knew he had to contact you.

After Abel has an opportunity to share, you thank him for coming to your office and express your genuine desire to help him decide on the next steps moving forward. You also affirm how difficult it feels to face rejection from his son. After processing further, Abel agrees to completing a safety plan and wants to restart regular counseling sessions. Following the session, you reach out to Dr. Lin Son, a trusted colleague, and consult about the session. Dr. Son affirms your choice of action but recommends Abel revisit the treatment hospital that provided his initial services. He recommends you call Abel with this suggestion and document the day and time of the call as well as Abel's response.

CASE OF ABEL (ENTIRE CASE IN CHAPTER 2)

SOAP SESSION NOTE

Client Name: Abel Tesfaye
Session Date: 11/4/2024
Session Number: 11

	Type of Session:		Nature of Contact:
X	Individual		Scheduled Appointment
	Group		Walk-in
	Couples	X	Emergency/Crisis
	Family		

Subjective: Client reported suicidal ideation after discovering negative comments from his son. He also reported means and a plan, specifically stating he would use the gun at his apartment in an abandoned field near his workplace. After discussing with clinician further, client reported he was no longer thinking of following through with his plan. Client expressed his appreciation for the clinician and asked if he could restart therapy.

Objective: Client was visibly anxious, seen by wringing his hands and rubbing them on his legs. His appearance was disheveled. He utilized previous cognitive distortions of all-or-nothing thinking regarding the worth of his life. Clinician used alternative interpretations and cognitive reframing to help client break his negative feedback loop.

Assessment:

Diagnosis: F33.2 major depressive disorder, recurrent, severe without psychotic features

Suicidal ideation: Present

Suicidal means: Present

Suicidal plan: Present

Suicidal intent: Active at start of session. Client reported intent decreased by the end of the session.

Client answered 4 out of 5 on the asQ Suicide Risk Screening Tool indicating high risk, so the asQ Brief Suicide Safety Assessment was administered. Client completed all areas of the assessment, and disposition was noted as "Patient might benefit from non-urgent mental health follow-up." No further evaluation necessary at this time.

Plan: Client has completed a suicide safety plan and wishes to reinstate therapy sessions. Clinician will consult with a colleague on any other courses of action.

Tara Pist, MEd

Clinician Signature

PATIENT SAFETY PLAN

Client: Abel Tesfaye

My triggers/warnings:

1. Negative feedback from loved ones
2. Failing at a work or school task/assignment
3. Letting my negative thoughts get to me

What I can do to distract myself:

1. Go for a run
2. Start a puzzle
3. Listen to worship music

People who can help distract me:

1. Bob @ work (555) 216-3982
2. Ed @ bike shop (555) 216-4692

People who I can ask for help:

1. Father Kidus (555) 603-4726
2. Ema (555) 782-3194

Professionals I can go to in a crisis:

1. Ms. Pist
2. Western Samaritan Hospital (555) 216-7373
3. National Suicide Hotline 988

How I can make my environment safe:

1. Sell my gun
2. Dispose of unused medication
3. Display Scripture-affirming messages around the house

Abel Tesfaye — Client

Tara Pist, MEd — Witness/Clinician

SOAP SESSION NOTE ADDENDUM

Client Name: Abel Tesfaye
Session Date: 11/4/2024
Session Number: 11

Additional information: After consultation with Dr. Lin Son, Clinician called client and recommended he return to the hospital where he had visited for his previous suicidal ideation. Client agreed this would probably be the best course of action and said he would go that afternoon. He asked to reschedule his next appointment with the clinician for 2 weeks after the original date, so November 25, 2024.

ADDITIONAL CRISIS CASE EXAMPLES

Below are additional case examples for the reader to reflect on and thoughtfully consider their responses to the questions that follow each example.

Case Examples: Adam

Part A

A clinician has been counseling Adam, a 52-year-old, White man, about marital issues. The client came to counseling at his wife's request. He was initially hesitant but has become active and engaged over time. He was forthcoming about his anger and how that impacted his marriage. He reported that he was not the best husband but that he thinks he is a good dad. The client identified areas for growth and made progress in meeting his treatment goals (reducing anxiety, reducing anger and frustration, regulating his nervous system, and improving communication). He was transitioning out of treatment and wanted to thank the clinician. He reports getting "a lot out of the sessions." At his last session, he gave the clinician tickets to a sporting event as a thank you. The tickets would be considered "expensive" but did not cost the client additional money (as he has season tickets). The tickets were for the clinician's favorite team, and the clinician would love to attend the event.

Question to ponder: Is this an ethical issue? Would you keep the tickets? Justify your answers. How and where should the clinician document the interaction/gift receiving?

Part B

Instead of presenting the tickets at the last session, the client dropped off a thank-you card that contained the tickets. This occurred after the client terminated services. He dropped the gift off with the receptionist. The client is no longer on the clinician's caseload.

Question to ponder: Does that change how and where the clinician would document that information? Explain your answer.

Part C

A month after receiving the gift, the clinician received a subpoena to go to court to testify on behalf of the client in a custody dispute. The client expects that the clinician will be helpful in court.

Questions to ponder: Does this information change how you would respond to the previous questions? If so, why?

Case Example: Jayde

Part A

Jayde is a 26-year-old biracial woman who has been attending counseling for 3 months. She is attending counseling for addiction issues and anxiety symptoms. Jayde reports that her substance use began after she was sexually assaulted (age 15). Jayde reported that she was assaulted by her uncle but will not provide a lot of detail about the situation. She reported that after the assault she began using alcohol and pills to help her feel numb. The amount and frequency of use increased, and despite trying to stop numerous times, Jayde has been unable to stop using. She reports reduced use but still engages in risky behavior at times. She does not meet the qualifications for inpatient addiction or mental health treatment. Jayde recently reported finding out that she is pregnant after having a "one-night stand" while she was drunk. She reports that the stress of her pregnancy has increased her alcohol use and that she secretly hopes that the alcohol will cause a miscarriage. This causes the clinician to have negative thoughts about the client. The clinician identifies as a Christian and is opposed to abortion. Because the clinician is having such an adverse reaction to the client, the clinician is debating her options: reporting the client for abuse of the baby/attempting to harm or abort her unborn child, telling the client how she feels about the situation, or referring Jayde to another clinician.

Questions to ponder: Does the clinician have to report the previous sexual assault? Are there ethical issues in this case? Explain your answers. How and where would you document the information related to this case?

Part B

You are a colleague of the aforementioned clinician, and she is telling you about the client's case. She is very upset and states that she "just needs to vent for a minute." She starts talking about the client's case and states that the client is "basically a killer and that it is not right for people to be irresponsible and then punish the baby for their actions." She reports that she has negative thoughts about the client and that she has been short with the client in the previous session. The clinician stated that she thinks it is because she "can't stomach the fact that she is being this stupid." She does not provide the client's name, but you are pretty sure that you know to whom she is referring. You recommend that she talk with her supervisor prior to seeing the client again.

Questions to ponder: Are there ethical codes by which you (the colleague) need to abide, related to the clinician's ethical behavior? How would you proceed? Would you document this interaction? If so, how and where? If not, provide justification.

Case Example: Alex

Part A

Alex is a 15-year-old teenage girl who identifies as African American. She has attended weekly counseling sessions for approximately 6 months. She is engaged in counseling, works toward meeting her treatment goals, and demonstrates good insight. At her most recent session, Alex reports being "scared" because she is having a "resurgence of suicidal thoughts—well, more like obsessions." She reports that she "has been thinking about it a lot" and even when she practices her coping strategies (singing, listening to positive music, journaling), she cannot stop her thoughts from turning to death. She indicated that she thinks about how she will die, why she should die, how the world would be better without her, and that no one would care if she died. She reports that she "mentally walks through how she could die by suicide" via overdose or jumping off of a bridge. Alex reports being hospitalized for 3 days approximately 2 years ago from a suicide attempt via overdose. She also admits to "a few" additional attempts that did not result in hospitalization. She stated that she "took pills and just woke up the next day and didn't tell anyone." Alex is estranged from her parents and is currently living with her aunt. Alex states that she feels bad because she knows that her parents are ashamed of her and that she is a financial burden on her aunt. When asked about her support system, Alex states that she does not have a lot of friends and tries to keep to herself at school. Alex reports that she does not fit in with other people in her community and cannot wait to move away from the small town. Alex is smart and has maintained a 3.7 GPA in school.

Questions to ponder: How would you assess Alex's risk of harm? Who would you tell about the information that Alex disclosed? How would you document the crisis information disclosed by Alex? What additional details would you obtain from Alex during the session?

REFERENCES

American Counseling Association. (2014). *2014 ACA code of ethics.* https://www.counseling.org/docs/

American Mental Health Counseling Association. (2020). *Ethical decision-making model.* https://www.amhca.org/viewdocument/amhca-ethical-decision-making-model

American Psychological Association. (2017). *Ethical principles of psychologists and code of conduct.* https://www.apa.org/ethics/code

Cottone, R., & Claus, R. (2000). Ethical decision-making models: A review of the literature. *Journal of Counseling and Development, 78,* 275–283.

Forester-Miller, H., & Davis, T. E. (2016). *Practitioner's guide to ethical decision making* (Rev. ed.). American Counseling Association. https://www.counseling.org/docs/ default-source/ethics/ practioner's-guide-toethical-decision-making.pdf

Knoll, J. L. (2019). Psychiatric malpractice grand rounds: The Tarasoff dilemma. *Psychiatric Times*. https://www.psychiatrictimes.com/view/psychiatric-malpractice-grand-rounds-tarasoff-dilemma

Ling, T. J., & Hauck, J. (2017). *The ETHICS model: Comprehensive ethical decision making*. VISTAS Online.

National Association of Social Workers. (2021). *Code of ethics of the National Association of Social Workers*. https://www.socialworkers.org/About/Ethics/Code-of-Ethics/Code-of-Ethics

Substance Abuse and Mental Health Services Administration. (2020). *National guidelines for behavioral health crisis care - A best practice toolkit*. https://www.samhsa.gov/sites/default/files/national-guidelines-for-behavioral-health-crisis-care-02242020.pdf

Stanley, B., & Brown, G. K. (2012). Safety planning intervention: A brief intervention to mitigate suicide risk. *Cognitive Behavioral Practice*, *19*, 256–264

Index

D

E

F

G

H

I

J

K

L

M

N

P

U

www.ingramcontent.com/pod-product-compliance
Ingram Content Group UK Ltd.
Pitfield, Milton Keynes, MK11 3LW, UK
UKHW050141280726
14058UKWH00006B/768